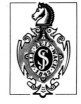

The Contribution of Acute Toxicity Testing to the Evaluation of Pharmaceuticals

Edited by
D. Schuppan, A. D. Dayan and F. A. Charlesworth

With 6 Figures and 21 Tables

Springer-Verlag
Berlin Heidelberg New York
London Paris Tokyo

Dr. Dietrich Schuppan
Manager, Medical and Scientific Affairs
Bundesverband der Pharmazeutischen Industrie e. V.,
Karlstraße 21, D-6000 Frankfurt am Main 1

Prof. Dr. Anthony D. Dayan
Director, DHSS Dept. of Toxicology
St. Bartholomew's Hospital Medical College,
Dominion House, 59 Bartholomew Close
GB-London EC1 7ED

Frances A. Charlesworth
Manager of Scientific Affairs
The Association of the British Pharmaceutical Industry – ABPI
12 Whitehall
GB-London SW1A 2DY

ISBN 3-540-15331-4 Springer-Verlag Berlin Heidelberg New York
ISBN 0-387-15331-4 Springer-Verlag New York Heidelberg Berlin

This work is subject to copyright. All rights are reserved, whether the whole or part of the material is concerned, specifically those of translation, reprinting, re-use of illustrations, broadcasting, reproduction by photocopying machine or similar means, and storage in data banks. Under § 54 of the German Copyright Law where copies are made for other than private use, a fee is payable to "Verwertungsgesellschaft Wort", Munich.

© by Springer-Verlag Berlin Heidelberg 1986
Printed in Germany

The use of general descriptive names, trade names, trade marks, etc. in this publication, even if the former are not especially identified, is not to be taken as a sign that such names, as understood by the Trade Marks and Merchandise Marks Act, may accordingly be used freely by anyone. Product Liability: The publisher can give no guarantee for information about drug dosage and application thereof contained in this book. In every individual case the respective user must check its accuracy by consulting other pharmaceutical literature.

Printing: Beltz Offsetdruck, 6944 Hemsbach/Bergstraße

Bookbinding: G. Schäffer, 6718 Grünstadt

2127/3140-543210

IFPMA Symposium

Geneva 30–31 October 1984

Organized by

Bundesverband der
Pharmazeutischen Industrie (BPI)
Frankfurt am Main

and

Association of the British
Pharmaceutical Industry (ABPI)
London

Sponsored by
International Federation of Pharmaceutical
Manufacturers Associations (IFPMA)
Geneva

With the support of the
European Federation of Pharmaceutical
Industries' Associations (EFPIA)
Brussels

Preface

The LD50 determination was originally devised in 1927 as a measure of acute toxicity and lethality for the standardisation and comparison of certain highly active, naturally occurring substances such as insulin and digitalis. Since that time it has become widely used as a means of providing a standardised measure of acute toxicity which is used as a basis for the classification of the potential hazards of chemicals and pesticides and as a starting point for the safety evaluation of pharmaceuticals and other products. This formal method appears to be very convenient in administrative terms, because it provides a "standardised" figure which can be used to classify a chemical. As a result, what was devised as a laboratory procedure for the purpose of bioassay, became a formal part of toxicity testing of candidate medicines and industrial chemicals. The official requirement became standard almost regardless of the other information available on the product and the inherent uncertainties of the test.

Since that time research has shown that the simplicity of the LD50 is illusory as both quantitative and qualitative findings are strongly influenced by the conditions under which the study is conducted. It has been realised that acute, single but high dose toxicity represents only a limited part of the biological data that are necessary to appreciate the effects of a new medicine. As the scientific attitude towards the test has changed, less reliance has been placed on the LD50 determination.

Lessening scientific interest in the classical LD50 determination has been reflected in moves by regulatory bodies to change their requirements. The pharmaceutical industry in the Federal Republic of Germany, the USA and the UK have expressed doubts about the value of the formal LD50 study. The IFPMA (International Federation of Pharmaceutical Manufacturers Associations) recognised that although the scientific and industry opinion had clearly changed over the last few years, the change in regulatory opinion is, of necessity, slower. It may not be possible for all industries to adopt similar forms of modified acute toxicity testing. The IFPMA therefore decided to hold an international seminar on the LD50 determination designed for regulators and scientists to meet and hear current views on acute toxicity testing.

The meeting at which these views were debated took place in Geneva in October 1984. Scientists from academia, regulatory institutions and industrial laboratories met and were able to discuss all aspects of the way in which an acute toxicity determination should be made for all types of products from medicines to industrial chemicals and some of the limitations to the methods. In almost all the formal papers and throughout the discussions, there was a theme on which there was general agreement – the classical LD50 test was no longer necessary as part of the development of a new medicine. Regulations are changing and in due course the administrative decisions and legal controls will reflect a corresponding shift in attitude. The scientific view is clear. We are pleased that the forum provided by the meeting enabled this group to reach such a consensus. Our thanks are due to the IFPMA for sponsoring the meeting and to the many other individuals and organisations that supported the meeting.

D. Schuppan
A. D. Dayan
F. A. Charlesworth

Contents

Preface VII

List of Contributers XI

Opening Remarks 1
G. FÜLGRAFF (Chairman)

I. Current Acute Toxicity Testing – How & Why?
G. FÜLGRAFF (Chairman)

Scope of Acute Toxicity Testing – Current Methodology 5
G. ZBINDEN

Use of Acute Toxicity Data for Pharmaceuticals 10
E. SCHÜTZ

Industrial Uses of Acute Toxicity Testing 20
G. J. A. OLIVER

Acute Toxicity Test Data –
Has It Any Relevance for the Management of Acute Drug Overdose in man? . 34
G. N. VOLANS

Acute Toxicology Viewed from the Pharmaceutical Industry 42
M. SCHACH VON WITTENAU

In Vitro Models for Acute Toxicity Testing 46
J. M. FRAZIER

II. Current Regulatory View on Acute Toxicity Testing
J. GRIFFIN (Chairman)

EEC/CPMP 55
R. BASS

Appendix 60

Single Dose Toxicity 61

A US/FDA View of Acute Toxicity Testing in the Evaluation
of Pharmaceuticals 65
L. M. Crawford

Current Regulatory View of Acute Toxicity Testing in Japan 74
M. Tezuka and A. Takanaka

Alternatives to Animals in Toxicological Assessment and Notifications 81
V. H. Morgenroth

III. Summary Reports of Group Discussions

Introductory Comments on Ethical Aspects of Acute Toxicity Testing 89
A. D. Dayan

Scientific Constraints on the Use of Acute Toxicity Testing 91
B. B. Newbould (Rapporteur)

Practical Constraints on the Use of Acute Toxicity Testing 93
J. M. Frazier (Rapporteur)

Regulatory Constraints on the Use of Acute Toxicity Testing 95
A. Steiger (Rapporteur)

IFPMA – A View on Acute Toxicity Testing in Relation to Pharmaceuticals . . 96
R. Arnold

Closing Remarks 99
G. Fülgraff (Chairman)

Sucject Index 103

List of Contributors

ARNOLD, R., Dr., International Federation of Pharmaceutical Manufacturers Associations (IFPMA), 67, rue de St. Jean, 1201 Geneva, Switzerland

BASS, R., Prof. Dr., Head, Drug Toxicology, Bundesgesundheitsamt, Postfach 330013, 1000 Berlin 33, Federal Republic of Germany

CRAWFORD, L. M., Dr., Director, Center for Veterinary Medicine, U. S. Food and Drug Administration, 5600 Fishers Lane, Rockville, Maryland 20857, USA

DAYAN, A. D., Prof. Dr., Director, DHSS Department of Toxicology, St. Bartholomew's Hospital Medical College, Dominion House, 59, Bartholomew Close, London EC1 7ED, Great Britain

FRAZIER, J. M., Prof. Dr., Department of Environmental Health Sciences, The Johns Hopkins University, 615 N. Wolfe Street, Baltimore, Maryland 21205, USA

FÜLGRAFF, G., Prof. Dr., Clausewitzstraße 8, 1000 Berlin 12, Federal Republic of Germany

GRIFFIN, J., Director, Association of the British Pharmaceutical Industry (ABPI), 12 White Hall, London W1, Great Britain

MORGENROTH, V. H., Dr., Organization for Economic Cooperation and Development, Chemicals Division, 15, Boulevard Amiral Bruix, 75016 Paris, France

NEWBOULD, B. B., Dr., Research Director, ICI Plc, Pharmaceuticals Division, Alderley Park, Macclesfield, Cheshire SK10 4TG, Great Britain

OLIVER, G. J. A., Dr., Acute Toxicity Section, ICI Plc, Central Toxicology Laboratory, Alderley Park, Macclesfield, Cheshire SK10 4TG, Great Britain

SCHACH VON WITTENAU, M., Dr., Pharmaceutical Manufacturers Association, Pfizer Central Research, Pfizer Inc., Eastern Pomit Road, Groton, Connecticut 06340, USA

SCHÜTZ, E., Dr., Head, Drug Toxicology, Hoechst AG/Außenstelle Kastengrund, 6234 Hattersheim, Federal Republic of Germany

STEIGER, A., Dr., Bundesamt für Veterinärwesen, Schwarzenburgstraße 161, 3097 Liebefeld – Bern, Switzerland

TAKANAKA, A., Dr., Chief, Pharmacologic Sciences, National Institute of Hygienic Sciences, Tokyo, Japan

TEZUKA, M., Department Director, Evaluation and Registration, Pharmaceutical Affairs Bureau, Ministry of Health and Welfare, Tokyo, Japan

VOLANS, G. N., Dr., Director, National Poisons Centre New Cross Hospital, Avonley Road, London SE14, Great Britain

ZBINDEN, G., Prof. Dr., Institut für Toxikologie, Eidgenössische Technische Hochschule, 8603 Schwerzenbach, Switzerland

Opening remarks

G. Fülgraff (Chairman)

The object of this international meeting of scientists from academia, industry and government is to describe current practice and to review the state of the art with respect to the assessment of acute toxicity of new chemical entities. The aim is to find out, if, where, and by what means the formal "LD50 test" can be modified or even replaced by other less stereotyped and more intelligent methods using fewer animals and/or different endpoints. Industry and regulatory practitioners are increasingly embarrassed and pressurised by animal protection associations which can substantially influence public opinion. A recent sample survey in the Federal Republic of Germany showed, for instance, that the number of those who are unconditionally against animal experiments has doubled in the past three years. It now amounts to up to 20%, and a further 60% approximately of the population is in favour of reducing and restricting experiments with animals. I suppose that the figures are similar in many other countries.

There are strong organised groups fighting against animal experiments in the United States, the United Kingdom, the Federal Republic of Germany and Switzerland, and the beginning of such movements in Scandinavia and Italy. In some countries, the question of animal experiments has become a political issue when new legislation on animal protection and animals in research is in preparation, for instance in the United Kingdom and in the Federal Republic. I remember well from the time that I worked in government, how difficult it was to convince even open-minded politicians and non-scientists of the sense and necessity for formal LD50 test. And I can imagine the discussions are not easy for politicians when they are confronted in their constituencies with single issue campaign groups fighting against animal experiments.

Now, at first glance, they always seemed to have ethics on their side. My own Minister of Health was an active and convinced member of the animal protection association and suffered from the fact that he could not do more to restrict animal experiments. I am sure that any step in the direction of avoiding or reducing animal experiments will be welcomed by the public. Therefore it fits well that an increasing number of scientists in academia, industry and government have during the past years expressed their doubts about the validity and ubiquitous requirement for the formal LD50 test. But, as is often the case, colleagues in industry feel that regulatory opinion changes too slowly, whereas colleagues in government agencies feel that it is industry which sticks to check-lists on formal grounds and does not want to abandon them in exchange for a more flexible and case by case approach. I feel that it is very worthwhile and merits recognition that IFPMA, the European Federation of Pharmaceutical Industries Association, the Bundesverband der Pharmazeutischen Industrie and the Association of the British Pharmaceutical Industry have joined together to sponsor this meeting, which brings together scientists from all sides to overcome their mutual prejudices, and, as it is said by the organizing committee, to consider new avenues to the subject of acute toxicity testing. I am convinced that the results of this meeting will find their way into industrial research practice as well as into regulatory requirements.

I. Current Acute Toxicity Testing – How & Why?

Scope of Acute Toxicity Testing – Current Methodology

G. Zbinden

Historical Background

Pharmacologists working in the early years of this century were mainly concerned with very toxic substances, such as cocaine, echitamine, chloroform, digitalis glycosides, dysentery toxin and insulin. As a consequence, mortality of laboratory animals must have been a frequently observed occurrence in their daily work. Thus, knowledge of the lethal dose was an essential prerequisite, without which the experimental analysis of the pharmacologic characteristics of a new chemical could not proceed [3]. Obviously, the information that a certain dose of a compound kills all animals, was of little practical value, since it did not indicate whether or not half the dose or a tenth of it would have the same effect. What was really needed was the knowledge of the "minimal lethal dose", i.e. that point on the dose-effect curve from where on mortality was to be expected [6].

It soon became apparent that the "minimal lethal dose" was also not a sufficiently defined endpoint, owing to the variation in susceptibility of individual animals. This was of little concern for drugs whose therapeutic and lethal effects were far apart, but it created considerable problems for compounds with a narrow margin of safety [3]. Moreover, the ill-defined "minimal lethal dose" was not suitable for substances that were not available in chemically pure form and for which the lethal effect was used for the purpose of biological standardization [6].

In order to obtain more relevant information about the lethal effect of a substance in a given population of laboratory animals, it was necessary to use several doses ranging from the "maximum tolerated dose" to the "certainly lethal dose", and to determine the percent mortality for each dose included in the experiment. It was found that each compound had a unique frequency distribution of the individual lethal doses, and that this distribution pattern was characteristic of the drug and the species and strain of laboratory animals used [4, 6].

It is unquestionable that determination of the lethal effects over the whole range of doses used, gives the most comprehensive information about the toxicological characteristics of a chemical substance. Therefore, it is surprising that the pharmacologists working in the twenties and the thirties were eagerly looking for ways to reduce this information to a single figure. In order to do this, the arithmetic mean, the mode or the median of the individual lethal doses could be calculated. For purely practical reasons, Trevan [6] selected the median lethal dose, termed it lethal dose 50%

(LD50), and with this proposal, he scored an immediate and lasting success. For Trevan's [6] own purposes, the standardization of biological substances, the determination of the LD50 was sufficient, because he always compared the test substance with a standard sample, and was not interested in the shape and steepness of the dose-effect curve. But those pharmacologists who uncritically adopted the procedure for the determination of toxicity of new chemicals sacrificed valuable information for the sake of simplicity provided by a single magical figure, the LD50 value.

Mortality is the most unequivocal of the quantal (all or none) responses in biology. Therefore, it is understandable that data generated in acute toxicity tests were seized eagerly by biostatisticians who used them to develop and validate the concept of the "bioassay". By straightening the S-shaped and sometimes kinked dose-mortality curves through mathematical transformations, statisticians facilitated the determination of "exact" LD50 values and simplified calculation of the steepness of the dose-effect curves. In addition, by attaching confidence limits to the LD50 values, they endowed them with an aura of scientific respectability. A further simplification was the introduction of graphical methods which made the evaluation of test results even easier [2].

Current Methodology

At present, acute toxicity tests are mainly conducted with mature rodents of both sexes, particularly mice and rats. Groups of 5 to 10 or more animals are treated with single doses expected to cause death in 10 to 100% of the subjects. The route of administration is that used in humans, and if this is the oral route, the test is often repeated with parenteral application. Doses are spaced logarithmically, and at least 4 to 5 dose levels are given. The experiments are rigidly standardized with regard to environmental and housing conditions, preparation and volume of application of the test material, size, age, strain and nutrition of the laboratory animals. Subjects are observed for at least 2 weeks or longer (usually 4 weeks) if the clinical status and body weight gain of the survivors indicate that complete recovery has not occurred. The number of dead animals at each dose and the time of death are recorded. These data are used to calculate the LD50 with 95% confidence limits. Details of the procedure are published in toxicological handbooks [1].

In recent years, much more emphasis has been placed on the observation of functional signs of toxicity [8]. First, a check-list approach was developed which permitted the recording of type, time of onset and duration of functional signs of toxicity, e. g. disturbances of central and autonomic nervous system functions, and of the cardiovascular, gastrointestinal and the respiratory systems. These evaluations are based on observational techniques with a simple scoring system (sign present or absent, sign mild, moderate or severe). More recently, objective and quantitative measurements of physiologic functions have been used, e. g. body temperature, locomotor activity, open field behavior, heart rate, and particularly for substances given by inhalation, rate of respiration.

Biochemical analysis of body fluids and haematological studies are rarely performed, but should be considered in special cases. Most standard protocols require autopsy, not only of spontaneously dying animals, but also of the survivors. Recording the weight of the major organs gives important additional indications about potential target sites for toxicity. Histopathological examination of the organs is rarely performed, but it should be considered for all organs showing distinct alterations on gross observation, but not for those with agonal changes such as fresh subcapsular hemorrhage and discoloration due to irregular distribution of the blood.

Scope of Acute Toxicity Testing

In the last 50 years, the problems related to acute toxic hazards of chemicals have dramatically increased in number and complexity. Animal safety data were deemed necessary for a large variety of chemicals, and the purposes for which the LD50 test was applied also multiplied. A list of the most important reasons for which LD50 tests are performed is presented in Table 1 [7].

Table 1. Purposes of Acute Toxicity Testing

Pharmacology and Toxicology
Determination of lethal dose for biological standardization of drugs
Detection of acute, hazardous effects
Identification of target organs and systems of toxicity
Determination of the therapeutic index of a new drug
Information on dose selection for pharmacological and repeated-dose toxicity studies
Information on bioavailability
Hazard assessment for drug combinations

Human Safety
Prediction of toxic and lethal dose in man
Prediction of symptomatology of human intoxication
Information on reversibility of acute toxic lesions
Hazard detection for risk populations (e.g. babies)
Information on usefulness of antidotes and other therapeutic measures

Governmental regulations
Integral part of registration dossier
Basic information for classification of chemicals in lists of poisonous substances

The current controversies pertaining to acute toxicity testing do not stem from the opinion that the data on hazardous effects of chemicals after high single dose administration to laboratory animals are useless for the evaluation of human safety, or that the many pharmacologic and toxicologic questions, summarized in Table 1, are irrelevant. What is debated is the question whether or not the test procedure with its main emphasis on determining an exact numerical value of the LD50, represents the most appropriate experimental approach. The most important aspects of current acute toxicity testing that are criticized are listed in Table 2.

Table 2. Major Criticisms of Current Practice of Acute Toxicity Testing

---
Test is used for purposes for which it is obsolete or poorly suited
Test is aiming at level of precision not required for most purposes
Test is needlessly performed with substances that pose no significant hazard of acute intoxication
Insufficient efforts are made to minimize the number of animals used and to obtain the maximum of scientific information from each subject
Insufficient efforts are made to eliminate or alleviate pain and anxiety of the animals

---

It is not the purpose of this introductory paper to identify those purposes of acute toxicity testing for which the conventional testing strategy is inadequate. Subsequent contributions will deal with this aspect in greater detail. Moreover, the subject has been treated in an earlier paper [7]. However, it appears necessary to discuss at least some of the bioethical aspects of the test procedure and the questions pertaining to animal welfare.

A test whose major end-point is death inevitably causes considerable hardship to at least some of the subjects. Therefore, it is essential that such an experiment is only done when an overwhelming interest for human protection can be demonstrated. The minimum number of animals necessary to achieve the goals of the test must be used, and the experiment must be conducted in such a way that a maximum of relevant information is gained from each subject sacrificed in the name of human safety.

Efforts must be made to reduce as much as possible stress, pain and anxiety of the laboratory animals. For example, substances known to be corrosive or causing marked local irritation should not be tested in concentrations that cause severe pain. It is desirable to start the tests with low doses that cause neither serious distress nor death. Subsequently, doses may be increased until the maximum tolerated dose or the minimum lethal dose is reached. This proposal is at variance with current practice which requires that all groups are dosed on the same day. This procedure may eliminate some day to day variations and saves time. But otherwise, it has no obvious advantage. However, it can lead to an excessive number of deaths, if in the process of dose selection the toxicity of the test compound is underestimated.

For many purposes, the maximum tolerated dose provides sufficient information, and the LD50 or the "certainly lethal dose" need not be determined [5]. This is particularly true for compounds with low acute toxicity, where a predetermined upper dose limit (e.g. 3 to 5 g/kg) must not be exceeded, even though no signs of toxicity and no deaths have been observed (limit test). If the treatment causes severe distress, the experiment must be terminated and the animals must be sacrificed.

Conclusions

For many substances introduced in the environment, knowledge of the hazards to humans and animals following acute exposure to large doses or high concentrations is of great importance. For this reason, experimental methods to determine the lethal doses and the symptomatology of acute intoxication have been developed for over 100 years.

The determinaton of the LD50 in small rodents is the most widely used procedure for this purpose. Unfortunately, pharmacologists and toxicologists have, for many years, concentrated their best efforts on obtaining a highly precise numerical value of the median lethal dose. In recent years, however, it has been recognized that knowledge of the signs of acute intoxication, the target organs of toxicity, the apparent cause of death and the probability of recovery from poisoning are of much greater importance for human safety than the availability of a numerical LD50 value determined with high precision [8]. Therefore, testing strategies have been revised and techniques providing a much greater spectrum of information on morbidity have been developed. In addition, heightened awareness of animal welfare has led to a revision of the test procedures and to the development of experimental protocols that require only small numbers of animals. Moreover, efforts are now undertaken to minimize pain and stress to the laboratory animals used in acute toxicity experiments.

References

1. Balazs T (1970) Measurement of acute toxicity. In: Paget GE (ed) Methods in Toxicology. Blackwell Scientific Publications, Oxford Edinburgh, pp 439–81
2. Litchfield JT Jr, Wilcoxon F (1949) A simplified method of evaluating dose-effect experiments. J Pharmacol Exp Ther 96: 99–113
3. Schlossmann H (1935) Toxizitätsbestimmungen, a Bestimmung der Dosis letalis. In: Abderhalden (ed) Handbuch der biologischen Arbeitsmethoden. Urban und Schwarzenberg, Berlin, pp 1714–1721.
4. Shackell LF, Williamson W, Deitchman MM, Katzman GM, Kleinman GS (1925) The relation of dosage to effect. J Pharmacol Exp Therap 24: 53–65
5. Tattersall ML (1982) Statistics and the LD50 study. Arch Toxicol (Suppl) 5: 267–270
6. Trevan JW (1927) The error of determination of toxicity. Proc Roy Soc 101B: 483–514
7. Zbinden G (1984) Acute toxicity testing, purpose. In: Goldberg AM (ed) Acute Toxicity Testing: Alternative Approaches. Mary Ann Liebert, New York, pp 3–22
8. Zbinden G, Flury-Roversi M (1981) Significance of the LD50-test for the toxicological evaluation of chemical substances. Arch Toxicol 47: 77–99

Use of Acute Toxicity Data for Pharmaceuticals

E. Schütz

Knowledge of the acute tolerance of food, natural substances and products manufactured therefrom has always been one of the most important resources and experience of mankind. It has actually permitted survival and in times of need the alleviation of pain, as well as the healing of wounds and diseases.

That is only one facet, however, as knowledge of the toxicity of various substances was soon used to put disagreeable people or competitors out of the way. This was probably the beginning of the first deliberately conducted toxicity tests. The lethal dose was tested in domestic animals – exposed sovereigns kept so-called "tasters" in order not to fall victim to poisoning.

For centuries the acute toxicity of vegetable, animal and active mineral substances was empirically determined before they were introduced as useful, therapeutic agents in folk medicine. Systematic toxicity tests only started at the beginning of modern drug development in the middle of the last century, with *Rudolf Buchheim* and *Oswald Schmiedeberg* as the initiators. In their time preparative and synthetic chemistry opened up the possibility of isolating active ingredients and taking the first steps for their chemical modification. These substances had then to be tested for their medicinal efficacy and usability. To that end pharmacologists had, just like today, to compare the efficacious dose with the harmful, lethal dose. Even at that time the diverse reactions of different animal species and the problem of extrapolation of the findings to man were known. Administration and observations in a few animals of different species were carried out personally by pharmacologists.

Let us now first look at acute toxicity tests as they were conducted by our early pharmacological colleagues. They actually served for many decades as the basis for assessing the safety of many drugs.

The most important journal for such investigations was the "Archiv für Experimentelle Pathologie and Pharmakologie" (Archives for Experimental Pathology and Pharmacology) published in 1873 by the pathologist *Klebs*, the internist *Naunyn* and the pharmacologist *Schmiedeberg*. To exemplify developments let us examine one volume every ten years, to see what is said about acute toxicity tests.

Johannes Fick, assistant to *Schmiedeberg* in Strasbourg in 1873, tested the toxicity of sparteine in a frog, a cat, and a rabbit. The latter were closely observed and the signs were meticulously recorded. After supplementary tests in an additional 8 frogs and 1 dog, *Fick* described the features of poisoning after administration of sparteine [7].

30 years later, at the Pharmacological Institute of the University of Tokyo, *Muto* and *Ishizaka* verified these findings, and through toxicity tests in 7 rabbits extended knowledge of the cause of death in cases of sparteine poisoning [15].

In 1881 in Strasbourg, *Vincens Cervello* investigated the pharmacological-toxicological effect of *paraldehyde*. 20 animals, namely 9 frogs, 8 rabbits, 2 dogs and 1 cat, were sacrificed in these tests [2].

Six years later, *Rudolf Cohn,* from 1887–1890 assistant to Geheimrat *Jaffe* at the Pharmacological Institute of the Royal Albertus-University of Königsberg i. Pr., characterized the toxic effect of *furfural* after tests in a few frogs, cats, rabbits and dogs [3].

In 1913, *Gröber,* of the Pharmacological Institute of the University of Berlin, at the time when *Arthur Hefter* was a full professor there, described the pharmacological-toxicological effect of *strophanthidin*. 13 frogs and 11 rabbits were used to determine its toxicity [11].

Those were the times of the most economical animal consumption in toxicity tests. They involved animals which were not bred for that purpose and were of the most varied state of health, age and breed.

The ability to isolate natural active ingredients, chemically to modify them and to obtain series of synthetic components was rapidly increasing during those years. It was necessary to standardize natural substances, such as cardiac glycosides, and later on hormones for clinical use, and to select from series of synthetic compounds the substance with the broadest therapeutic range. Consequently, it was essential to standardize toxicity tests and initially this concerned above all acute toxicity testing. Mathematical methods allowing reliable comparison of the toxicity of various batches or derivatives had to be developed. *Trevan* in 1927 was the first to describe a practicable method for the standardization of digitalis, in which the mean lethal dose, the "LD50", served as the comparative value [20].

During the following years and up to the present innumerable mathematical and statistical methods have been developed in order to indicate the LD50, always with a higher accuracy. Normally, at least five male and/or female animals per dose have been employed. At least three but as rule more doses have been used. Initially, it was obligatory also to determine on the one hand the dose which killed no animal and on the other hand that which would kill all animals.

The trend to investigate large series of chemical compounds for acute toxicity in a comparable way did not have its origin in the pharmaceutical industry. It was the rapid *development of the chemical industry as a whole* which entailed the *dissociation of industrial toxicology from pharmacology*. In 1925, the year of foundation of IG-Farbenindustrie, the Institute of Industrial Hygiene was set up by BASF in Ludwigshafen. In Germany, this was the beginning of the independent development of toxicology in industrial research. At a university level, toxicology was first introduced at the Pharmacological Institute of the University of Würzburg, headed from 1920 to 1945 by *Ferdinand Flury* [13]; a member of the Flury family is here today.

A look at the first volume of *Spector's* "Handbook of Toxicology", Vol I: "Acute Toxicities" [18], published in 1956, shows that by far the largest proportion of the 2120 enterally and parenterally tested substances listed there were investigated for reasons of industrial toxicology and not on pharmaceutical grounds. The determination of the lethal concentration, the LC50, which is analogous to the determination of the LD50, for a further 243 substances by inhalation, was done almost exclusively for reasons of industrial toxicology.

Efforts towards increasing the comparability of LD50 values soon resulted in the breeding of laboratory animals with increasing genetic *homogeneity*. This led finally to the extreme demand of *Spiegel* [19] to breed laboratory animals "pro analysi".

At that time it was hardly asked whether the constant striving for higher accuracy in animal experimentation by use of inbred strains was entirely relevant for man. Growing knowledge of "pharmacogenetics", which is reflected in the differing reactivity of individuals to certain active ingredients, should have given food for thought.

As long as the effects of substances are to be compared with one another, and as long as they must be *classified,* investigations in homogenous animal specimens are inevitable, if economically efficient work is to be safeguarded. But, if only for financial reasons, such large series of substances should no longer be tested in this traditional way and with so many animals.

Consequently, methods have been sought to limit animal consumption in acute toxicity tests for such purposes. *Deichmann* and *Leblanc* [4] already described in 1943 a method for the determination of an "approximate lethal dose" with about *six* animals. *Lichfield* and *Wilcoxon* [14] published a statistical method, which enables the confidence limits to be indicated no matter what values they might actually have in such tests, which are subject to very different influences. This could be done without having to determine an LD50 and an LD100. Their technique contributed at that time to saving many animals.

In pharmaceutical research *Paul Ehrlich* [6] introduced the term "chemotherapeutic index" [16] for determination of the therapeutic range of a new active ingredient. It is calculated as the ratio that the maximum tolerated dose bears to the minimum curative dose in case of single administration.

Meanwhile the statistical processing of pharmacological-toxicological test results had constantly gained in importance. Soon, the "LD50" also included data on confidence limits, values which were readily listed in publications, together with other pharmacological parameters and physico-chemical constants as exemplified in Table 1.

The importance attached by pharmacologists or toxicologists to LD50 data in the development of drugs could be readily understood from the published values. Unfortunately several unexpected drug intoxications occured in the meantime. Because of them, in 1955, the American FDA published [8] an "experimental program for appraising the safety of chemical components of foods, drugs and cosmetics". In 1959 the FDA [9] issued a revised version of the "Appraisal of the safety of chemicals in foods, drugs and cosmetics" with detailed instructions for the determination of LD50 values.

In 1956, thalidomide, which had appeared non-toxic in acute tests, was introduced into therapy as "Contergan" [12]. It caused neurological damage in cases of chronic use and unexpected but dramatic malformations in neonates. This accident, which

Table 1. Pharmacological parameters and physico-chemical-constants

	Compound			C 3080	V 346	C 5123	C 5327	C 5124	C 3061	C 3049	C 3192	C 3181
Chemistry	Substitution of the phenyl ring			phenyl	phenyl	phenyl	CH$_3$-phenyl	CH$_3$-phenyl	Cl-phenyl	Cl-phenyl	BuOOC-phenyl	phenyl
	Side chain			—NH·OC—CH$_2$—N(C$_2$H$_5$)$_2$	—N·OC—CH$_2$—N(C$_2$H$_5$)$_2$ / CH$_2$	—N·OC—CH$_2$—N(C$_2$H$_5$)$_2$ / C$_2$H$_5$	—NH·OC—CH$_2$—N (pyrrolidine)	—N·OC—CH$_2$—N (pyrrolidine) / C$_2$H$_5$	—NH·OC—CH$_2$—N(C$_2$H$_5$)$_2$	—N·OC—CH$_2$—N(C$_2$H$_5$)$_2$ / CH$_3$	—N·OC—CH$_2$—NH·C$_3$H$_7$(n) / Bu	—N·OC—CH$_2$—N (piperidine) / Bu
	Solubility at 20° C	g$_0$	mg/cm^3	~650		238		490		87,3	580	
Local Anesthesia	Rate of increase	a	min	58,3	51	57	54,8	64	56,9	45,3	70,5	60,3
	Duration of anesthesia 1% solution	b	min	40,5	18	18	38	3,25	6,7	10	36	8
	Difference of paresis	c	%	0,05	0,1	0,4	0,13	0,35	0,35	0,3	0,44	0,65
	Lower effect level	k$_o$	%	0,5	0,7	0,73	0,5	0,95	0,89	0,8	0,6	0,875
	Concentration with 1 h duration of anesthesia	k$_1$	%	1,4	2,3	2,1	1,49	2,43	2,55	3	~1,4	~2,37
	Latency period	t$_L$	min	1,6	2	3,5	2,5	5,5	6	7	2,5	3
	Failure percentage	U	%	<3	15,3	24	5	20	33	12	22	50
	Specific activity of anesthesia	s	min/mg	8,58	5,36	5,74	8,05	4,96	4,7	4,16	8,65	5,07
	Corneal anesthesia 2% solution	t$_o$	min	0	0	0	0	0	7,50	0	>24 h	>24 h
Toxicity	Duration of poisoning	t$_T$	h	4	2,7	1,9	4	1	6	2	5	8
	LD$_{50}$ Mouse sc.	d$_M$	mg/20 g	16,5	13,4	3,4	17,4	1,75	16	7	56,5	75
	LD$_{50}$ Mouse ip	d$_p$	mg/kg	280	200	100	262,5		375			
	LD$_{50}$ Rat ip	D$_M$	mg/kg	430	260	140	448	63,5	318	220	260	480
	Safety Quotient	pT= d$_M$/k$_i$		11,8	5,77	1,62	11,7	0,72	6,27	2,33	40,3	31,6
Irritation	Degree of corneal irritation	R$_o$	Grad	0	0	0	1	1	1	1	>4	>4
	Chemical irritation (pH of turbidity)	K$_p$	pH-Grad	7,1	8,21	8,55	7,55	8,9	6,3	9,04	5,3	5,4
	Concentration of medium irritation (rat)	P$_M$	%	1,4	2,1	1,9	1,55	2,15	0,63	1,7	0,135	0,16
	Tissue compatability quotient	pR= P$_M$/k$_i$		1	0,91	0,9	1,04	0,885	0,247	0,566	0,096	0,067
Total Evaluation	Absolute area of anesthesia	I$_A$		83,5	46,6	49,4	78,8	33,3	35,7	33,7	80,4	38,6
	Total anesthesia compatible area	I$_T$		336	221,5	67,3	345	11,9	238	106	730	598
	Tissue compatible area of anesthesia	I$_R$		31,1	30,5	26,1	35,1	21,3	<0	12,8	<0	<0
	Total utility	Z		105	82,2	42	110	16	0	37	0	0

became apparent in 1961, had the most serious consequences for the pharmaceutical industry. Manufacturers of drugs and of other chemicals were forced extensively to reform their toxicological testing. From 1961 legislators in almost all countries throughout the world issued toxicological test provisions which regulated amongst other things the determination of acute toxicity. These provisions are constantly being updated.

In 1962, the European Society of Drug Toxicology was founded. In 1963, the German Pharmacological Society [5] issued recommendations on the pharmacological-toxicological testing of new drugs. It recommended an acute toxicity test with a sufficiently large number of animals for determination of the LD50 with the possibility to draw dose-effect curves for the administration of the drug via different routes. Orientation tests were to be conducted in two additional species, including the dog.

In 1980 *Zbinden* [1] and his colleagues collected the various international test guidelines for drugs. On the basis of these guidelines almost all states required acute toxicity tests in two rodent species, with a number of animals that allows calculation of the confidence limits of the LD50, and an approximate value in one non-rodent species. As a rule, dogs and in some instances rabbits are considered as non-rodents. Normally, two routes of administration, the oral and a parenteral route are demanded, one including the therapeutic route. The follow-up period in most cases is fixed; usually for 1 week, but occasionally up to 2 weeks of the disappearances of the symptoms of intoxication.

It is now legally required that a new drug or a new drug combination can only be supplied even for a single administration to man after several animal toxicity tests have been conducted. In almost all cases this makes it necessary to measure the enteral and parenteral LD50, values with confidence limits in at least two animal species, and that at least orientation findings in larger animals must be available. The inclusion of several animal species in acute toxicity tests actually increases safety by increasing the likelihood of identifying the species producing the features of intoxication comparable to those in man, despite possible differences in metabolism. To achieve this is one of the essential reasons underlying the implementation of acute toxicity determinations. The physician must know what side effects to take into account and what symptoms will be apparent in case of overdosage, whether unintended or envisaged with suicidal intent. It is the only way to develop antidotes in due time or to elaborate therapeutic proposals for their invention. Since the official regulation of the toxicological testing of new chemicals and drugs by legal provisions or binding recommendations has come about, it can no longer be clearly deduced from publications which acute toxicity tests the expert himself has considered necessary and which tests were only conducted in order to comply with legal provisions.

Nevertheless, it is still interesting to look at the publications of the representative German language magazine "Arzneimittel-Forschung" ("Drug Research") published since 1951 in relation to LD50 determinations and their breakdown by individual species (Table 2).

These data are strongly influenced in individual years by the fortuitousness of publication of values for long series of homologues, whose "therapeutic index" was to

Table 2. LD50 Determinations published during 1953–83 in Arzneimittelforschung, Verlag Editio Cantor, D-7960 Aulendorf

Year of Publication	Total LD 50s reported	Rat/Mouse	Rabbit/Hamster Guinea Pig	Dog/Cat Monkey
1953	17	12	3	2
1954	184	174	10	–
1955	258	243	10	5
1956	132	121	8	3
1957	253	230	19	3
1958	826	782	28	16
1959	513	494	13	6
1960	359	342	14	3
1961	455	402	5	48
1962	164	150	14	–
1963	209	184	21	4
1964	351	341	2	8
1965	290	261	25	4
1966	213	202	8	3
1967	459	425	18	16
1968	361	339	8	14
1969	318	290	11	17
1970	220	174	35	11
1971	409	386	15	8
1972	320	295	11	14
1973	228	205	10	13
1974	271	243	10	18
1975	297	267	21	9
1976	259	219	28	12
1977	433	419	7	7
1978	158	137	15	6
1979	142	119	13	10
1980	261	238	16	7
1981	324	301	12	11
1982	101	93	4	4
1983	178	162	7	9

be compared. Altogether this made LD50 determinations an easy test, which was readily delegated to younger colleagues or co-workers. However, appraisal of the findings from acute toxicity tests requires a good measure of experience. Experienced pharmacologists and toxicologists have always known of the dependence of LD50 values on the quality and state of the laboratory animals, as well as on manifold external circumstances. Some of the most important of these factors being:

In 1968, *Schütz* [17] stressed the great importance of the orally administered volume in rodents and the relativity of LD50 values obtained by this route. His co-worker *Fuchs* [10] investigated the marked influence of many additional parameters on the numerical value of the LD50. These and other references, particularly those from the working group of Zbinden [21] in Zurich about the incorrect understanding of LD50 values alone, would probably not have been sufficient to initiate reforms in this field. The pressure of public opinion, which had previously demanded more and

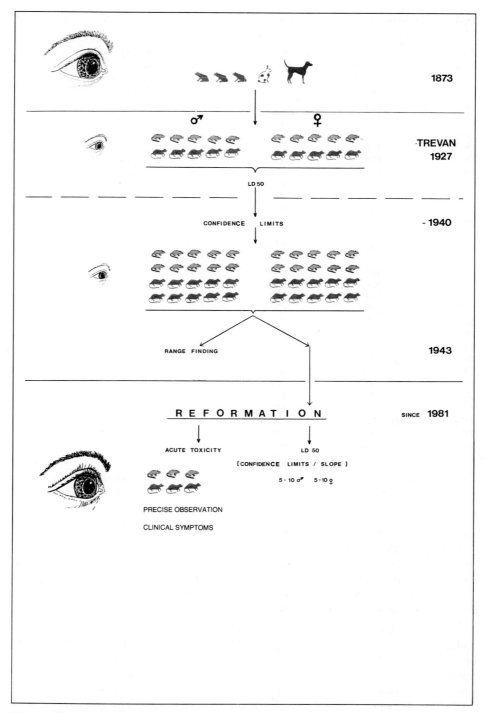

Fig. 1. Historical development of acute toxicity testing

more intensive animal tests in response to the pressure of drug incidents, was required to point out the undesirable increase in animal consumption which had meanwhile occurred. The LD50 rapidly became one of the irritant words, constantly used by active antivivisectionists in a well meant but uninformed way when demanding the total abolition of this type of test. Unfortunately, that demand has also been thoughtlessly supported by some expert colleagues. The debate on acute toxicity tests is a challenge for toxicologists to stand their ground between scientific requirements and feasibility on the one hand and the pressure of the public (or properly speaking the published) opinion on the other.

It must be clearly stated here that acute toxicity tests, occasionally including determination of the LD50, are the most important first attempts of toxicologists at the beginning of safety tests relating to new substances with a so far unknown action. In this connection, knowledge of the acute toxicity of a drug is of direct benefit for the protection of the consumer, i.e. the patient. The question is only how this test should be designed in order to take the justified demand of reasonable animal protection sufficiently into account without suffering an unacceptable loss of the findings. We must state that for most indications there is not yet an alternative to experiments in living animals for acute toxicity tests.

Great importance must be attached, as we have always emphasized, to intensive observation of laboratory animals after administration of toxic doses by well trained staff members. The period of observation of the animals, which at the beginning of the tests are usually juvenile, should be extended until the body weight curves of all surviving animals show an upward tendency. The ideal condition of former times, that experienced experts personally carried out the administration and intense follow-up observations, cannot always now be realized (Table 3).

Table 3. Factors which can influence the results of the Acute Toxicity Tests

Species	Cage size
Strain	Season
Sex	Climatic conditions
Age	temperature
Body weight	humidity
Diseases	air pressure
Parasitization	
	Formulation
Quality of feed	Quality of vehicle
Feeding condition (fasted/nonfasted)	Bioavailability of test substance
Maintenance	Administered volume
single	Rate of application
group	Handling during application

Figure 1 represents the historical development of acute toxicity tests. We should make it our concern to use as few animals as possible and only as many as are absolutely necessary in tests, and to investigate and observe them as intensely as is feasible.

It is most desirable from various points of view that the international endeavour of harmonization and of mutual acceptance of acute toxicity data required by regulatory authorities will be successful.

References

1. Alder S, Janton C, Zbinden G (1981) "Preclinical Safety Requiremens in 1980". Inst. of Toxicology, Swiss Federal Institute of Technology and University of Zurich
2. Cervello V (1883) „Über die physiologische Wirkung des Paraldehyds und Beiträge zu den Studien über das Chloralhydrat". Arch. exper. Path. Pharm. *16*, 265–290
3. Cohn R (1893) „Über die Giftwirkungen des Furfurols". Arch exper Path Pharm *31*, 40–48
4. Deichmann WB, LeBlanc TJ (1943) "Determination of the Approximate Lethal Dose with about Six Animals" J Industr Hyg Toxicol *25:* 415–417
5. Deutsche Pharmakologische Gesellschaft (1963) „Mitteilung des Vorstandes der Deutschen Pharmakologischen Gesellschaft und der Kommission zur Aufstellung von Richtlinien für die Prüfung neuer Arzneimittel". Arch exper Path Pharm *245*, Heft 1, Geschäftliches S 17–31
6. Ehrlich P and Hata S (1964) „Chemotherapie der Spirillosen", Berlin 1910; quoted after M Schneidermann et al "Toxicity, the Therapeutic Index, and the Ranking of Drugs". Science *144*, 1212–1214
7. Fick J (1873) „Über die Wirkung des Sparteins auf den thierischen Organismus". Arch exper Path Pharm 1, 397–413
8. Food and Drug Administration (1955) Dir of Pharmacology and Food, "Appraisal of Safety of Chemicals in Foods, Drugs and Cosmetics". Food Drug Cosmetic Law Journal *10*, 679
9. Food and Drug Administration (Topeka, Kansas 1959) Dept of Health, Education and Welfare, "Appraisal of the Safety of Chemicals in Foods, Drugs and Cosmetics"
10. Fuchs H (Ingenieurarbeit, Frankfurt (M)-Höchst 1976) „Durchführung und Auswertung enteraler sowie parenteraler akuter Toxizitätsversuche unter besonderer Berücksichtigung präparatunabhängiger Faktoren"
11. Gröber A (1913) „Über Strophanthidin". Arch exper Path Pharm *72*, 317–330
12. Kunz W, Keller H and Mückter H (1956) „N-Phthalylglutaminsäure-imid – Experimentelle Untersuchungen an einem neuen synthetischen Produkt mit sedativen Eigenschaften". Arzneimittel-Frsch *6*, 426–430
13. Lindner J (Aulendorf i Wttbg 1957) „Zeittafeln zur Geschichte der pharmakologischen Institute des deutschen Sprachgebietes"
14. Lichfield jr JT and Wilcoxon F (1949) "A Simplified Method of Evaluating Dose-effect Experiments". J Pharmacol exper Therap *96*, 99–113
15. Muto K and Ishizaka T (1903) „Über die Todesursache bei der Sparteinvergiftung". Arch exper Path Pharm *50*, 1–10
16. Schneidermann MA, Myers MH, Sathe YS and Koffsky P (1964) "Toxicity, the Therapeutic Index and the Ranking of Drugs". Science *144*, 1212–1214
17. Schütz E (1968) „Über die akute orale Toxizitätsprüfung". Arzneim Frschg *18*, 466–469
18. Spector WS (Editor) (Philadelphia and London 1956) "Handbook of Toxicology, Vol I: "Acute Toxicities"
19. Spiegel A (1963) „Über das Versuchstier 'pro analysi'". Dtsch med Wsch *88*, 1203–1206
20. Trevan IW (1927) "The Error of Determination of Toxicity". Proc Roy Soc London, Ser B, *101*, 483
21. Zbinden G and Flury-Roversi M (1981) "Significance of the LD50-Test for the Toxicological Evaluation of Chemical Substances". Arch Toxicol *47*, 77–99

Discussion following Prof. Zbinden and Dr. Schütz

The importance of careful observation of animals in tests was re-emphasized. Alterations in behaviour and other clinical signs could give a considerable amount of information about effects on the somatic and autonomic nervous systems. Similarly, appearances at autopsy and often the weights of organs were all valuable pointers to the sites and possible mechanisms of damage.

Prof. Zbinden

It is often believed that no relevant information is available when toxicity studies are first undertaken, but this is very rarely the case. In practice, most people are working with a series of compounds and they already know the major characteristics of those compounds, for example, whether they are convulsants or hepatotoxins, etc. If you have no idea at all about the compound, then you must first do a broad screen.

It is clear that the simple observational studies are procedures that can be done well, but which require very experienced people to do them. I believe that there is a machine which measures the mobility of an animal. You put the animal in and then the machine will calculate the LD50 by recording the moment when the animal ceases to move. That of course is one extreme. At the other extreme, as Dr. Schütz' paper clearly shows, these is the pharmacologist who looks at the compound in great detail and identifies the major targets of toxicity. I believe that all animals should be autopsied and that the most important thing is the gross observations. The pathologist should identify those organs which are likely to be damaged and those which show agonal changes. Quite often weighing the organs gives helpful information. An organ of normal weight which looks normal is likely not be badly damaged. I do not believe that clinical chemistry is much help in an acute study. Histology is rarely helpful except when the organ is clearly changed.

Dr. Warren

Does Professor Zbinden feel that studies of behavioural signs would be helpful in evaluating possible toxic effects?

Prof. Zbinden

They are very important. It is relatively easy to look at effects on the autonomic nervous system. There are simple ways of detecting most autonomic effects in animals. Whether or not more elaborate behavioural studies are necessary is questionable. It is worthwhile to study mobility, and simple parameters, such as body temperature, could be measured. More elaborate neurological behavioural tests should not be necessary.

Industrial Uses of Acute Toxicity Testing

G. J. A. OLIVER

Introduction

Several thousand new chemicals are synthesised each year, many of which will add to those already used in commerce. There is both a moral and legal obligation on the chemical industry to ensure that the risk of adverse effects to human health and the environment is minimal in order to competently satisfy society's rightful demands for safety. Generally, this obligation is met by toxicity experiments using animal species to provide surrogate data from which risk to human health may be determined.

Society's requirement for protection and safety is accompanied by a parallel concern for the welfare and humane use of animals in scientific experiments, including toxicity experiments.

This apparent conflict of interests has directed the attention of those concerned with chemical (both industrial and pharmaceutical) safety evaluation to current requests for and the supply of specific toxicological data. Are relevant questions concerning chemical safety being asked and are attempts to answer them being made in the most appropriate way, particularly with respect to the use of animals?

Criticism of toxicity studies has focussed particularly on acute toxicity tests and often on one specific experimental end-point, the median lethal dose or LD50 value. The acute toxic properties of a chemical are often equated with this single parameter. This practice has frequently been criticised, since an LD50 value alone does not represent the full range of acute toxic effects that may occur, and also because it has long been seen to be of limited use as a biological reference point except in very well defined circumstances [3, 7, 29, 33].

Individual scientists, industrial organisations and government authorities as well as animal welfare groups have called for re-evaluation of current requirements for LD50 values, and reconsideration of those regulatory guidelines which recommend and detail experimental protocols from which these values can be derived [2, 5, 8, 17, 31].

The purpose of this paper is to:
1. review the uses of acute toxicity data for industrial chemicals
2. discuss the use of lethality data and LD50 values
3. review acute toxicity procedures with respect to the total number of animals that need to be used.

The major theme of this paper concerns optimizing use of animals and any lack of reference to alternative models or *in vitro* systems should not be misconstrued to indicate their dismissal. The European Chemical Industry Ecology and Toxicology Centre (ECETOC) has instigated a task force which is reviewing the use of acute toxicity studies and alternatives to animal models; the findings of this working party, representing the views of the European Chemical Industry, will be published in early 1985 [11].

Definition of Acute Toxicity

Acute toxicity is defined as the adverse biological effect(s) which result(s) from short term exposure, i.e. following a single dose or an exposure not exceeding 24 hours. The observed acute effects may ensue rapidly or may be delayed in onset; they may be temporary or persistent. For many industrial chemicals and pesticides it has been shown that the most relevant route of exposure in the workplace or when crop spraying is either through skin contact and/or by inhalation if the material is volatile or forms a respirable atmosphere. Other less usual routes may be relevant – for example, some chemicals express a high systemic toxicity after exposure to the eye only [1].

An experiment to determine the acute toxic potential of a substance should generate, on a dose-response basis, information on the clinical signs or nature of intoxication, the onset, duration and severity of these effects together with an indication of the target organs (Fig. 1). From the various data (assessment of bodyweight, body functions and appearance, the macroscopic condition of internal organs at necropsy,

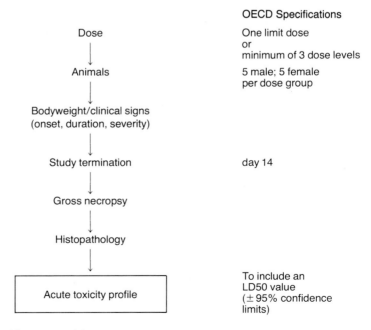

Fig. 1. Outline protocol for acute toxicity assessment

and in some cases microscopic examination of tissues) a composite picture may be drawn of the acute systemic toxic potential of any material.

For some purposes of acute toxicity testing an indication of the lethal dose range is necessary, and as such the mortality incidence forms part of the overall appraisal.

However, it is appropriate to state clearly the following two points:
1. it is not necessary to derive a precise LD50 value in order to obtain the lethal dose range;
2. a LD50 test (where only the median lethal dose is determined and all other information is ignored) is not the same as an acute toxicity test (as described above).

Many misconceptions have arisen purely from the erroneous interchange of these two terms (toxicologists being as guilty of this as anyone else) – it is easier to say "LD50" than "acute toxicity test".

Industrial Chemicals

In the context of this paper, the term "industrial chemical" refers to "non-pharmaceuticals" i.e. pesticides, organic and inorganic chemicals, intermediates, dyestuffs, solvents, surfactants, polymers, oils, biocides and additives. This selection reflects the author's own laboratory's experience rather than providing an exhaustive list.

Industrial and pharmaceutical chemicals have similarities and differences which are relevant to the approach to and significance of acute toxity assessments (Table 1).

Table 1. Characteristics of pharmaceutical and industrial chemicals

	Pharmaceuticals	Industrials	
		Pesticides	Others*
Biologically active	By design	By design	Incidental
Pharmacology/ mechanism of action	Mammalian	Non-mammalian	No information
Toxicology	Extensive	Extensive	More limited but increasing
Human exposure	Voluntary	Involuntary	Involuntary
Human symtomatology	Regular feedback	Irregular feedback	Irregular feedback

* Some industrial materials, eg. biocides, are more analogous to pesticides in many respects.

Pharmaceuticals and pesticides have common features in that they are selected because they possess a specific biological activity, albeit in different target species. To ensure that their biological activity is selective for the precise target, novel pesticides, in the early phase of their discovery and development, are usually assessed for their acute toxic potential. High mammalian toxicity may invalidate further progress.

Unlike pharmaceuticals, no prior knowledge of probable mammalian pharmacology is usually available for industrial chemicals prior for toxicity testing. Since acute toxicity studies tend to be the first scheduled, this reinforces the need for such assessments to be as general and comprehensive as practicably possible.

Human exposure to industrial chemicals is largely unintentional, being involuntary or accidental. The widespread and less easily controlled use of pesticides has resulted in mandatory, prolonged and extensive development programmes to ensure efficacy and safety. For pesticides, the acute toxicity testing phase represents only one part of a detailed toxicological assessment. This provides a contrast to many other industrial compounds, where acute toxicity tests may constitute the only evaluation of systemic toxicity.

Legislation in the USA and Europe regarding premarketing and pre-manufacture notification of new chemicals is rapidly changing this imbalance in the scope of regulatory toxicology.

A major aim of the toxicologist is to assess the probable effects of chemicals in man. Feedback from human exposure is essential if toxicological models and procedures are to be critically examined, modified and refined. Compared with pharmaceuticals, there is a paucity of accurate data regarding human exposure to industrial chemicals. Significant advances continue to be made in terms of occupation hygiene and workforce monitoring to provide information additional to that obtained from accidents and poisoning cases.

Uses of Acute Toxicity Testing

The main purpose of acute toxicity testing in the chemical manufacturing industry is to assess toxic potential in order to evaluate possible human hazard and to provide information that can be used to safeguard human health (Table 2). The majority of industrial chemicals are not intended for human contact. They will be used for their specific technical purpose irrespective of their toxic profile, if it is feasible to ensure adequate containment during normal manufacture and use. A knowledge of the acute toxic potential is necessary for the recommendation of appropriate working or use conditions. This is achieved by compiling labels and hazard data sheets, by recommending handling procedures and safety clothing, and even by influencing the design of chemical plant. Despite these precautions accidents occur and toxicity information is required then to assist the medical services.

In meeting the above demands the full range of dose-dependent acute toxicity symptomatology, referred to earlier, is essential. Since the maximum dose may not be

Table 2. Purposes of acute toxicity studies for industrial chemicals

1. To determine toxic potential, hazard evaluation, and protection of human health
2. For registration/notification
3. For classification, labelling and packaging
4. For antidote development
5. To determine the hazard of combined exposure
6. To provide information on bioavailability
7. To provide information for multiple dose toxicity tests

controllable in an accidental exposure, it is important to know the possible lethal dose range and accompanying agonal signs of toxicity. In most circumstances precise estimation of the lethal dose is unnecessary.

Toxic effects which are not peri-lethal may be of equal importance. For example, many aromatic amino and nitro compounds are used as essential intermediates in the manufacture of dyestuffs, drugs, pesticides and other chemicals. These compounds may cause cyanosis, due to methaemoglobinaemia, which may be apparent at doses significantly below a lethal dose. Certain pesticides may exert effects on motor activity and gait at doses divorced from the lethal dose. Such events cannot be ignored in recommending handling precautions, setting exposure conditions or advising medical personnel.

The process of hazard evaluation and the setting of safety standards have been incorporated internationally into various laws and other requirements. These regulate the manufacture, transportation and use of pesticides and other chemicals in relation to registration, notification, classification, labelling and packaging [18]. The majority of these use the LD50 value as the principal currency of acute toxic potential. The LD50 value forms the basis for the assignment of a chemical to a toxic class or category. Typical criteria for the classification of a substance are shown in Table 3. Although all are based on LD50 values, the range which denotes the toxic category varies for chemical types and uses, and between nations.

In general there is a requirement to provide data on one species (usually the rat) and two dose routes for industrial chemicals and for two species (at least) and three dose routes for pesticide products. Legislation for either chemical type does not require toxicity data in dogs or in primates.

Since it is not a "biological constant", the utilization of a precise LD50 value as a reference point for hazard classification has been questioned [21, 27]. However, the *status quo* is that industry provides LD50 values with 95% confidence limits to ensure appropriate classification and thus enable authorised trading.

In addition to the more commonly voiced reservations, there are indications that the data are under- and over-utilised. Although 95% confidence limits are required, how often is their significance considered? A 95% confidence limit is a statement of

Table 3. Criteria for the classification of substances

	Category	LD50 absorbed orally in rat mg/kg	LD50 absorbed percutaneously in rat or rabbit mg/kg	LD50 absorbed by inhalation in rat mg/litre (4 h)
Health & Safety Executive, UK (18)	Very toxic	25	50	0.5
	Toxic	25 to 200	50 to 400	0.5 to 2
	Harmful	200 to 2000	400 to 2000	2 to 20
Environmental Protection Agency (13)	I	50	200	0.05
	II	50 to 500	200 to 2000	0.05 to 0.5
	III	50 to 5000	2000 to 5000	0.5 to 5
	IV	5000	5000	5

the precision of the data set obtained, not an indication of a narrow range around a mean value. Thus, two compounds could have an LD50 value of 100 mg/kg but 95% confidence limits of 20 and 500, or 99 and 101 respectively (Table 3). For the first example, there is a possibility that the true value is 20 or 500. It is questionable, however, that these two compounds would be differentiated on classification grounds; both would be categorized according to their mean LD50 value.

Singular consideration of and over-reaction to the LD50 value can have significant commercial consequences. For example, it is impossible to register pesticides in certain parts of the world if the rodent LD50 value is equal to or less than 50 mg/kg – irrespective of the amount of supporting toxicological information. This example illustrates the need for a more enlightened approach to the interpretation of acute toxicity information, and the limitation of strict dependence on a precise LD50 value is supported by scientists, just as much as those concerned about animal welfare and commercial interests.

Less frequent reasons for acute toxicity testing are shown in Table 2. Antidote development is most relevant to pesticide usage. The probability of identifying an antidote is highest if the mode of toxic action is known. This in turn would suggest that specific physiological, biochemical or other end-points and not simply lethality should be measured in relation to the development and the effectiveness of any treatment.

Synergism or potentiation of toxic effects from joint exposure to two or more chemicals is obviously of relevance to risk assessment. Again, this usually relates to pesticide mixtures. Assuming that the acute toxic profiles of the independent active ingredients is know, a limited dose experiment with the mixture for comparative purposes may be appropriate. This might require a knowledge of the lethal dose ranges, but need not rely on comparison of precise LD50 values.

An indication of the bioavailability of industrial compounds is usually restricted to comparison of the relative absorption from two or more dose routes. For example, a chemical of low oral toxicity may be highly toxic by a parenteral route which may be relevant to hazard evaluation. This information is required by most authorities for pesticide registration. Whereas it may be relevant to know the lethal dose range, a precise LD50 value is unnecessary.

In other circumstances, e.g. for a specified dose route, when the bioavailability of an active ingredient from different formulations is required, then it is more appropriate scientifically to measure blood concentration kinetics for a full and accurate assessment of absorption to be made.

Lastly, single-dose studies often provide the first step along the road to multi-dose experiments. Although it may be advantageous to know the approximate lethal dose, a precise LD50 value is not necessary. It is less common for an experiment to be performed solely as a prelude to a repeated dose study. For many industrial chemicals single dose acute toxicity studies are the only ones ever performed; repeated dose studies are rarely commissioned.

Experimental Protocols, LD50 Values and Animal Numbers

There is no practical alternative to animals at present for comprehensively assessing acute toxic potential. For this purpose, animals should be used humanely and with an economy of numbers. Overt suffering and death and the pursuit of unnecessary precision should be minimised by appropriate protocol design.

Two positive approaches, which have resulted in a reduction in the use of animals, have been made in the regulatory field through the harmonisation of testing guidelines by the OECD [26], and the general acceptance of limit dose studies.

The basic OECD protocol is described in Figure 1. If no animals (from a group of 5 males and 5 females) die at a specified limit dose then no further testing is necessary. This has reduced animal numbers in acute toxicity studies considerably, since most substances are of low toxicity. A retrospective survey of data from the Central Toxicology Laboratory (CTL) showed that over two-thirds of test substances were of low toxicity and therefore fell into the single dose limit range (Fig. 2). A more logical integration of guidelines and classification systems is needed if limit doses are to have maximum effect in reducing experimental animal numbers, since the selected limit doses do not always relate to the classification schemes employed. For example, the oral limit dose in the EEC VIth Amendment [13], equivalent USA legislation [20] and OECD [26] guidelines is 5000 mg/kg. However, in the EEC, LD50 values in excess of 2000 mg/kg are not used in determining the lowest toxic category [12, 19] (Fig. 2). Therefore, international consistency in the selection of toxicity classes coupled to a single limit dose would avoid unnecessary additional testing of materials destined for sale both in the USA and the EEC.

Many experimental details of the OECD guidelines remain flexible. However, where limit doses are not invoked, there is a specific requirement for a minimum of three dose levels, and five animals of each sex for each of the dose groups. Consequently, there is a minimum requirement for 30 animals. It is often necessary to

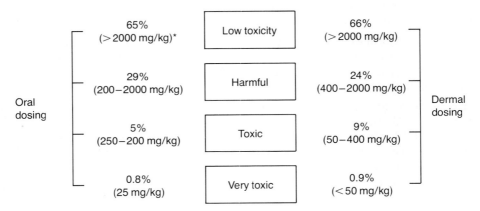

*figures in parenthesis represent the LD50 values characterising each toxicity class

Fig. 2. CTL survey (8 year period) of toxic categories following acute oral and dermal dosing studies (RAT)

precede such a study with a preliminary or pilot experiment to ascertain pertinent spacing of dose levels. If the initial data do not allow derivation of an LD50 value and 95% confidence limits, then additional dose groups may be necessary. From our own experience with the OECD protocol, approximately 30–50 animals, on average, will be used to provide the required data.

Where studies are not intended to meet regulatory requirements, protocol design is at the discretion of the toxicologist or study director. It should not be assumed, therefore, that "LD50 protocols" are routinely employed where the acute toxicity of industrial chemicals is being assessed.

An analysis of protocol types employed at CTL over a two-year period indicates that two-thirds of acute studies were range-finding experiments, which utilised between 4 and 12 animals in total, i.e. 2 animals per sex and up to 3 fixed but spaced dose levels (Fig. 3).

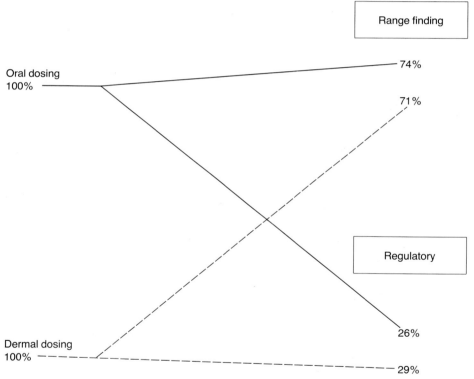

Fig. 3. Types of acute toxicity protocol employed at CTL (all other details are as outlined in Fig. 1)

These experimental designs provide data sets for translation into human hazard assessments for compounds which will be handled only within the company, e.g. pre-development pesticides, intermediates, low volume substances and various laboratory research chemicals. An estimate of the lethal dose range is determined, but not the precise LD50 value.

The combination of small numbers of animals with detailed clinical observations at frequent intervals, together with the optional use of additional specific measurements of homeostasis can often permit more detailed analysis of toxic effects [22]. This is a particularly useful approach for materials expected to possess biological activity, such as pre-development pesticides of novel structure, and has been shown to be effective in the selection of drugs for further development [15, 16].

If the purpose of an acute toxicity study is to derive an LD50 value, several publications have indicated that this can be achieved by using less than the 5 animals per group recommended in OECD guidelines (Table 4), thus enabling large savings in animal numbers.

Table 4. Comparative details of various acute toxicity protocols

Protocol	Total no. animals (males & females)	No. dose groups (of each sex)
1. OECD	30–50	3–5
2. Limit dose	10	1
3. Range-finding* (CTL)	4–12	3
4. Modified LD50 tests		
(Schütz & Fuchs 1982)	16–24	4–6
(Lorke 1983)	26	7
"Up-and Down" Test (Dixon, 1965; Bruce, 1984)	12–20	6–10

* No LD50 value derived

Following a retrospective analysis of 170 studies in rodents (five per sex per dose), Schütz and Fuchs [28] concluded that three animals per group provided LD50 values of a similar precision. If the dose groups were committed in a sequential way, such that the result of the initial dose was taken into account in setting the rest, then 2 animals per group would be sufficient in most cases. Tattersall [30] reached a similar conclusion.

Lorke [23] described a protocol where a maximum of 13 animals of each sex would provide estimates of LD50 values. An initial experiment, using three fixed dose levels with 3 animals per dose group, is used as a sighting procedure for up to 4 remaining dose levels with 1 animal per dose group.

In the "up and down" method [4, 10] a single dose is given to one animal. If the animal survives for 2 days, the next dose is given and is increased by a fixed factor until the original outcome is reversed. The dose for each successive animal is adjusted up or down depending on the outcome for the previous animal. Bruce recommends that after the first reversal of the initial result approximately 5 more animals are dosed to achieve a precise LD50 value. Although fewer animals are used than in a conventional OECD protocol, deaths delayed beyond 2 days disrupt the procedure. In addition, if the initially selected dose level is distant from the LD50 value then more animals may be needed to "home in" to the appropriate dose range. The sequential nature of the protocol also prolongs the experiment which may present logistical problems in the laboratory.

In addition to other aspects of experimental design it must be emphasised that selection of the appropriate statistical method of data analysis may influence the total number of dose levels and therefore numbers of animals used [6]. Weil [32] has highlighted the merits of the moving average method. This may have advantages over the more commonly used probit method in any experiment where only one intermediate mortality ratio exists between the 0% and 100% mortality dose levels. In contrast to probit analysis, the moving average method is compromised if dose levels are not equally spaced or if group sizes vary.

From both the toxicological and statistical viewpoint, it may be more advantageous to have a large number of dose groups with a small number of animals per group than vice versa.

In summary, there are a number of approaches which allow a full examination of dose-related acute toxic effects and precise LD50 determination but which use fewer animals than are recommended in OECD guidelines. It follows, therefore, that an immediate saving in animal numbers would be possible if all regulations relating to industrial chemicals, and which currently recognise the acceptability of the OECD guidelines, allowed flexibility in the numbers of animals per dose group.

Criteria for Toxicity Classification and LD50 Values

The bureaucratic reliance on the LD50 value as a cornerstone of hazard classification is pervasive and deeply entrenched. In the preceding discussion the use of more animals than necessary in deriving an LD50 value represents the quantitative aspect of today's debate on the use of animals. There is also a qualitative aspect. Irrespective of the exact protocol, wherever a precise LD50 value is derived, more animals will be given a lethal dose than in an experiment designed to determine only an approximation of the lethal dose range.

This represents a qualitative misuse of animals. However, to correct this, it will be necessary to replace the reliance of classification systems on an overprecise numerical value. The mechanism for allocation of chemicals to toxic categories must be revised. Fixed dose range procedures have been proposed as a possible way forward [5].

Animals are dosed at one of three fixed dose levels (Fig. 4). If survival at one level is more than 90%, with no evident sign of toxicity, dosage is increased by a factor of ten. If it is less than 90%, dosage is decreased by the same factor. Ultimately, a pre-set level is found that allows more than 90% survival and which specifies the classification. An average of 10 to 20 animals would be used. A claimed advantage is that at no time is the objective of the study to cause death of the animals, the toxicologist's decision to increase the dose level being guided by the signs of "evident toxicity" as much as by percent mortality.

Using the above approach a retrospective survey of 153 compounds indicated broad agreement of classification based on conventional LD50 protocols. A prospective

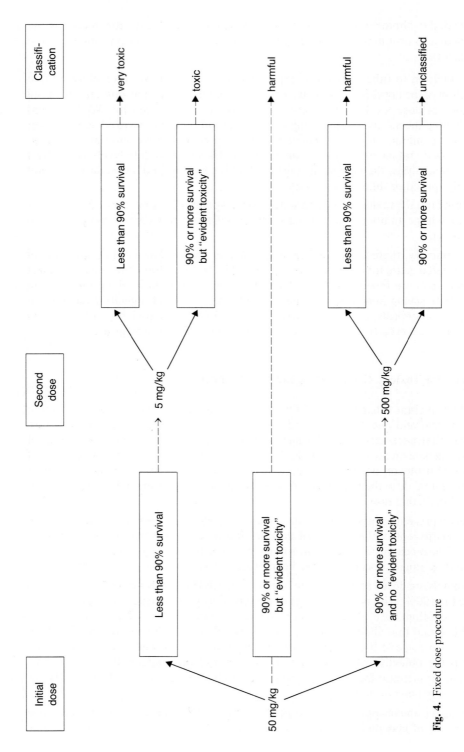

Fig. 4. Fixed dose procedure

comparison of the fixed dose range procedure and regulatory protocols is currently being organised to compare the quality and utility of the acute toxicity data produced by both approaches. Several toxicology laboratories in the United Kingdom have indicated their intention to participate.

The fixed doses suggested in the British Toxicology Society proposal have been selected to provide information that can be transcribed into the existing European classification system. As already stated these classification systems are not internationally consistent. Extra dose levels may be needed to give complete "regulatory cover" to chemicals destined for worldwide marketing. This is not always known when a test is commissioned. Unless a fixed dose range procedure accounted for all regulatory possibilities, a degree of retesting may result.

Reference or Orientation Protocols

Various retrospective data set appraisals have indicated that in general there is little difference between the sexes in terms of the expressed acute toxic profile [4, 9, 25, 28]. In many cases, therefore, it would be appropriate to determine the toxic profile in one sex first. A single or limited number of reference or orientation doses, targeted against this initial information, would suffice to provide relevant information for the other sex.

A similar argument can be used in other circumstances, e.g. species comparisons or formulation comparisons. Whilst it is fully acknowledged that a primary aim is to identify the unexpected through comprehensive assessment, in many cases this reference approach would be appropriate. Independent of the protocol design, this would contribute to a reduction in the numbers of animals used.

Summary and Conclusions

The need for acute toxicity assessment is fully recognised in the manufacture, development, and use of industrial chemicals. Criticisms are lodged essentially against the wrongful emphasis placed on the precision of particular data viz LD50 values.

LD50 values have been incorporated as the basic reference unit for internationally established regulations impinging on most facets of an industrial chemical's existence. This is the reality and undoubtedly the recognition and acceptance of a single parameter, the harmonisation of basic protocols and the implementation of limit doses have reduced the numbers of animals that might otherwise have been used for acute toxicity testing. In the regulatory sphere, the LD50 value is now being proposed as one of the basic units on which to construct directives for the categorisation of preparations [24]. Thus various protocols are being considered which utilise mathematical manipulations of the LD50 values of the separate components of formulations and preparations to establish a toxicity classification. Ironically, these directives are an attempt to minimise the need for additional acute toxicity studies on formulations and preparations.

The elimination of regulatory adherence to the LD50 value as a numerical index of toxicity will depend on constructive proposals and wide-ranging acceptance of practical alternative procedures for ranking toxicity and for classification procedures. This should be actively promoted and encouraged, but it would be naive to underestimate the difficulties to be surmounted in achieving such progress internationally.

As an interim position a relaxation of OECD guidelines in relation to the number of animals per dose group would have an immediate effect in terms of the total numbers of animals used in acute toxicity tests, without any loss of qualitative or quantitative data. In principle, this should be readily acceptable to all member countries of OECD which have endorsed the spirit of flexibility in the guidelines which state that each toxicity study should represent "... a scientific exercise" and not "... a set of stereotyped tests to be conducted in a routine" [26].

Overall, the climate is right for a major reconsideration of the perspective of acute toxicity data in relation to its uses for all industrial chemicals.

Finally, concentration on the LD50 issue should not distract attention and resources from other scientific aspects of acute toxicity evaluation – improving methodology, maximising the extraction of pharmacological, biochemical and physiological information and the pursuit of any additional systems that will improve the toxicologist's ability to predict human toxic effects in the most scientific, humane and cost effective manner.

References

1. Anon (1984) Chem Reg Rep *8*, 333
2. Bass R, Günzel P, Henschler D, Konig J, Lorke D, Neubert D, Schütz E, Schuppan D and Zbinden G (1982) LD50 versus acute toxicity. Critical assessment of the methodology currently in use. Arch Toxicol, *51*, 183–186
3. Brown VKH (1983) Acute toxicity texting. In: Animals and Alternatives in Toxicity Testing. Eds Balls, Riddell an Wordern, Academic Press, pp 1–16
4. Bruce RP (1984) An up-and down procedure for acute toxicity testing. In press
5. British Toxicology Society (1984) A new approach to the classification of subtances and preparations on the basis of their acute toxicity. A report by the British Toxicology Society Working Party on Toxicity. Human Toxicol *3*, 85–92
6. Chanter DO and Heywood R (1982) The LD50 test: some considerations of precision. Toxicology Letters *10*, 303–307.
7. Dayan A (1983) Complete programme for acute toxicity testing – not only LD50 determination. Acta Pharmacol Toxicol *52*, 31–51
8. Dayan AD, Clark B, Jackson M, Morgan H and Charlesworth, FA (1984) Role of the LD50 test in the pharmaceutical industry. The Lancet, 555–556.
9. Depass LR, Myers RC, Weaver EV and Weil CS (1984) Alternative Methods in Toxicology. Vol 2. Acute Toxicity Testing: Alternative Approaches. May Ann Liebert Inc, Publishers, New York
10. Dixon WJ (1965) The up-and-down method for small samples. J Am Stat Assoc *60*, 967–978
11. ECETOC Monograph N^0 6 (1985) Acute toxicity tests, LD_{50} (LC_{50}), determination and alternatives. Brussels
12. EEC VIth Amendment (1983) Directive 79–831, Annex VI, Part II B
13. EEC VIth Amendment (1984) Directive 79–831, Annex V
14. Environmental Protection Agency (1984) Federal Register *49*, (188), 37979
15. Fowler JSL, Brown JS and Bell HA (1979) The rat toxicity screen. Pharmacol & Therapeutics, *5*, 461–466

16. Fowler JSL and Rutty DA (1983) Methodolical aspects of acute toxicity testing, particularly LD50 determinations: present use in development of new drugs. Acta Pharmacol Toxicol, *52*, 20–30
17. Griffin JP (1981) Referring to the paper by Zbinden & Flury-Roversi. Arch Toxicol, *49*, 99–103
18. Hayes WJ (1982) Principles and Methods of Toxicology. Raven Press
19. Health & Safety at Work (etc) Act (1984) The Classification, Packaging and Labelling of Dangerous Substances Regulations 1984. No. 1244
20. Environmental Protection Agency Health Effects Test Guidelines (1982) EPA 560/6–82–001 (PB82–232984)
21. Hunter WJ, Lingk W and Recht P (1979) Intercomparison study on the determination of single administration toxicity in rats. J Assoc Off Anal Chem, *62*, 864–873
22. Irwin S (1962) Drug screening and evaluative procedures. Science (NY) *136*, 123–128
23. Lorke D (1983) A new approach to practical acute toxicity testing. Arch Toxicol, *54*, 275–287
24. Martens M, Mosselmans G, Fumero S, Jacobs G and Lafontaine A (1984) Some thoughts on a possible regulatory approach at EEC level on the classification and labelling of dangerous preparations. Reg Tox Pharmacol, *4*, 134–145
25. Müller H and Kley HP (1982) Retrospective study on the reliability of an "approximate LD50" determined with a small number of animals. Arch Toxicol, *51*, 189–196
26. OECD Guidelines for Testing of Chemicals (1981) Section 4: Health Effects. Test Guidelines, Nos 401, 402, 403
27. Schütz E (1969) On acute oral toxicity tests. Amer Perf Cosmet, *84*, 41–44
28. Schütz E, Fuchs H (1982) A new approach to minimising the number of animals used in acute toxicity testing and optimising the information of test results. Arch Toxicol, *51*, 197–220
29. Sperling F (1976) Non-lethal parameters as indices of acute toxicity: inadequacy of the acute LD50. In: New Concepts in Safety Evaluation. Eds Mehlmann MA, Shapiro RE, Blumenthal H, John Wiley and Sons, New York, London, Sydney, Toronto. pp 177–191
30. Tattersall ML (1982) Statistics and the LD50 study. Arch Toxicol Suppl, *5*, 267–270
31. Überla K and Schnieders B (1982) In reference to the paper by Bass et al. Arch Toxicol, *51*, 187
32. Weil CS (1983) Economical LD50 and slope determinations. Drug and Chem Toxicol, *6*, 595–603
33. Zbinden G and Flury-Roversi M (1981) Significance of the LD50 test for the toxicological evaluation of chemical substances. Arch Toxicol, *47*, 77–99

Acute Toxicity Test Data – Has It Any Relevance for the Management of Acute Drug Overdose in man?

G. N. VOLANS

Introduction

When a new drug is released for use in man, it should be assumed that sooner or later there will be cases of acute overdosage. These will occur sooner when the drug is an oral hypnotic, analgesic or antidepressant and thus very liable to be used as a means of self-poisoning; they will occur later when the drug is a parenteral agent and thus only liable to overdosage if there is an error in calculating the dose. Other drugs will present overdose problems with a frequency that is between these two extremes, depending upon their use, route of administration, frequency of prescription and ratio of toxic to therapeutic effects. It thus behoves both the manufacturer and the Poison Control Centres (PCCs) to prepare from the outset for the possibility of acute poisoning by a new drug. In this paper, I would like to present an account of how our PCC collates information and prepares advice on the presentation and management of drug overdosage and to demonstrate that acute toxicity data from animal tests contributes very little of value to this work.

The Role of a Poison Control Centre

The primary function of all PCCs is the provision of an emergency 24-hour information service to assist in the diagnosis and management of acute poisoning incidents. There are, however, other important functions served by such centres (Table 1) and

Table 1. The Functions of a Poison Control Centre (PCC)

1. Provision of information which can help directly in the management of acute poisoning in man. Increasingly, PCCs are becoming involved also in the assessment and management of suspected subacute and chronic poisoning in man
2. Provision of a consultative clinical service for advice on management and also for transfer/treatment of poisoned patients
3. Provision of a reference laboratory with a service commitment for the urgent and non-urgent biochemical analysis of drugs and poisons to be used in assisting the diagnosis and clinical management of poisoned patients; in evaluating the toxicity of particular chemicals and also in determining the use and value of treatment methods [20]
4. The collation and evaluation of data relevant to poisoning in man. This includes the important monitoring function now known as "Toxicovigilance" [9, 16]
5. Participation in measures intended to prevent poisoning including education of the public [18]
6. Training and education of doctors and other health service personnel in all aspects of poisoning in man [19]

most major centres in Europe and the U.S.A. are active in all these roles, either as a direct part of the PCC or in close collaboration with other departments.

If acute toxicity test data has any relevance for the management of acute poisoning in man, it should be demonstrable in the working of the information services. If it does not, the evidence against its value should be found from the clinical, laboratory and epidemiological activities.

Information Collection/Collation/Provision

Each PCC works with a specialist database which may take several forms but which is generally collated in a way designed to enable rapid response to the most common problems referred to that centre. In the London centre, for example, our in-house, firstline database is a self-generated, "Poisons Index" currently used in hard copy but capable of transfer, at least in part, to a computerised system.

Table 2. Scheme for Poisons Index Entry

Identification:		Toxicity Assessment:	
Type of Product	– intended use	Toxicity	– in man – in animals (if nil else)
Contents	– most toxic ingredients	Symptoms	– in man (or animals) – and time course
Description	– identification – dose calculation	Management	– supportive or specific – use of laboratory analyses
Manufacturer	– for further information		

Each entry in this index is divided into two parts, as shown in Table 2. The first part serves for product identification and calculation of dose whilst the second assesses toxicity and advises on management. For drugs, collation of this information is usually much easier than for other chemicals since much of what is needed will have to be generated in the application for a product licence. Table 3 summarises the main questions asked and the additional background information from which it is planned, where necessary, to monitor the first case reports of overdosage using our own version of a selective monitoring scheme. It can readily be seen that acute animal toxicity tests play only a small part in this database and that in all cases the animal data is considered "second best". This situation can be explained firstly by the failure of attempts to extrapolate from animal data to man and secondly by the successful development of a human case file which is used for toxicity assessment.

Table 3. Poisons Index Entries

Information required on new drugs
1. *Trade* and *Approved* names
2. *Pharmacological Group*/Intended use (Therapeutic Group)
3. *Formulations* and *identification* (N.B.: Sustained release preps.)
4. *Contents* – in order of expected toxicity
5. *Dose* – contained in each formulation
– maximum in therapeutic use (adult and child)
– pack sizes
6. *Toxicity* – in *man:* range of fatal doses/maximum dose survived
– or in *animals:* acute toxicity data
7. *Symptoms* – type and duration in man (or animals)
8. *Suggested Treatment* and source – by analogy
– from animal studies
– from human studies

Essential background for monitoring new drugs
1. Laboratory methods for analysis of drug in biological fluids
2. Pure sample as standard for establishing the method
3. Pharmacokinetics in man (or animals)
4. Toxic effects in first overdose reports (or observed in acute animal toxicity tests)

Comparison of Oral LD50 Data with Experience in Man

To illustrate the failings of the LD50, I will use examples from non-steroidal anti-inflammatory drugs (NSAIDs) and antidepressants.

Table 4 lists the rat oral LD50s for a range of NSAIDs. The most striking observation is that the safest molecules appear to be aspirin and ibuprofen. Clinical experience, however, does not accord with this since aspirin is well known to cause deaths in man in doses which are not difficult to take [11], whilst the largest overdoses of ibuprofen recorded in over 14 years' clinical use failed to produce serious toxicity in man, even at plasma concentrations over twenty times peak therapeutic levels [3].

Table 4. NSAIDs Acute Toxicity Tests

Rat Oral LD_{50} (mg/kg)

Substance	Sex	LD_{50}	95% Confidence Limits
Diclofenac	M	240	195– 294
	F	226	186– 274
Acetylsalicylic Acid	M/F	2170	1870–2510
Ibuprofen	M/F	1600	– –
Ketoprofen	–	101	– –
Indomethacin	–	12	– –
Naproxen	–	543	– –
Phenylbutazone	M	608	538– 687
	F	660	581– 764
Mefenamic acid		750	– –

Sources: RTECS
   Menassé *et al*, 1978. Scand. J. Rheumatol.

Further examination of these data suggests that the NSAIDs listed all have similar degrees of toxicity. This is not the case in man, however, since although most appear relatively safe in overdose, phenylbutazone can produce severe toxicity and death (Table 5) whilst mefenamic acid frequently causes convulsions (Table 6) [2].

Table 7 compares the oral LD50 in rats and mice for the antidepressants. Again, there are obvious failings since this does not suggest that subsequent clinical experi-

Table 5. Symptoms of Phenylbutazone Poisoning

Mild Poisoning

Nausea, abdominal pain, drowsiness

Severe Poisoning

Early Onset Upper abdominal pain, nausea, vomiting, haematemesis, diarrhoea, restlessness, dizziness, coma, convulsions (more prevalent in children) hyperpyrexia, electrolyte disturbances, hyperventilation, alkalosis or acidosis, respiratory arrest, hypotension, cyanosis, oedema, electrocardiographic abnormalities, cardiac arrest

Late Onset (2–7 days) Acute renal failure, increased values for liver function tests, followed by jaundice, electrocardiographic abnormalities, cardiac arrest, blood dyscrasias (anaemia, thrombocytopenia, leucopenia, or leucocytosis), hypoprothrombinaemia

Table 6. Symptoms occuring in mefenamic acid poisoning 1980–81 (patients aged 12 years and over) n = 58; Males 9 (17%); Females 45 (83%)

Age Range (Years)	No. of Cases	None	Symptoms	
			Convulsions	Symptoms other than convulsions
12–20	31	9	15	7
20–30	17	5	6	6
30 and over	4	3	1	–
Adult (age not specified)	2	2	–	–
Total	54	19 (35%)	22 (41%)	13 (24%)

Table 7. Antidepressants Acute Toxicity Tests

Substance	Oral LD$_{50}$ (mg/kg)	
	Mice	Rats
Amitriptyline	305	–
Dothiepin	320	450
Desipramine	500	385
Lofepramine	2500	1000
Maprotiline	660	760
Mianserin	380	1700 (M) 925 (F)
Nortriptyline	370	–
Nomifensine	400	430
Trimipramine	640	–

Table 8. Symptoms in Overdose from Tricyclic
Antidepressants (TCAs) Maprotiline, Mianserin and Nomifensine

Symptoms	TCAs %	Maprotiline %	Mianserin %	Nomifensine %
Coma	33.5	26	4.8	7.6
Drowsiness	39.3	56	38.1	38
Convulsions	12.7	30	0	0
Sinus Tachycardia	19.6	16	7.1	15.4
Depressed Respiration	5.7	8	0	0
Hypotension	6.3	4	2.4	0
Death	3.6	4	0	0

ence would demonstrate that mianserin and nomifensine are a great deal safer than the tricyclic antidepressants when taken in overdose in man (Table 8) [4]. Table 7 is also notable for the apparent lower toxicity of lofepramine as compared to the tricyclic antidepressants including its active metabolite, desipramine. This observation is being used to promote lofepramine, and is supported by studies in animals and in man, which suggest that the desipramine formed from lofepramine does not reach the same high levels found after metabolism of imipramine [7, 8]. It remains to be seen if this is supported in overdose cases, although the preliminary observations are encouraging [10].

Monitoring Human Drug Overdose Reports

It would not be difficult to produce further evidence to support the argument against the value of the LD50 for assessment of drug toxicity in man, It is, however, more important to consider the alternative sources of information. Volunteer studies of acute drug intoxication are, of course, largely outside normal ethical practice. Nevertheless, useful information can occasionally be gained directly or indirectly from Phase I studies, as in the case of naproxen, where dose ranging studies led to the investigation of its pharmacokinetics in doses up to eight times those subsequently recommended for therapy [17]. These observations suggested that naproxen would be of low toxicity in acute overdose and this has subsequently been confirmed in cases of deliberate self-poisoning [2].

Of greater importance than the limited volunteer studies are the data that can be collected on actual cases of drug overdosage, both accidental and deliberate, as they are reported to PCCs [9]. At our centre, for instance, we received telephone enquiries on over 35,000 cases of suspected poisoning during 1983, approximately half of which related to drugs. In all cases, a record of the enquiry is made, including details of the enquirer, the patient, the drug, symptom and treatment given so far. For selected cases, we undertake laboratory analyses for drugs either to assist in diagnosis and management or to assess toxicity [20], and we also seek information on the outcome. These case data are considered essential to the proper function of the service, and we continue to refine our monitoring techniques [9, 15, 21]. Most recently, we have established a computerised file for our case reports, which now gives us the ability to perform searches on a number of parameters but, most importantly, enables us to assemble reviews of human overdosage with particular substances, in response to clinical need, rapidly and comprehensively [5, 6].

The Future

In making my case against the value of LD50, I would not like it to be thought that I see no role at all for acute animal toxicity tests. Some assessment of the order of toxicity of a drug is still needed before it is used in man, and I believe that the current scientific debate on alternative tests, such as that prepared by the British Toxicology Society [1] should eventually lead to the official recognition of more cost-effective tests. Additionally, I would encourage further development of animal tests where physiological or biochemical evidence of the toxic effects is investigated, as in the study of ECG changes in rats given antidepressants [13].

At the same time, there is scope for further development of overdose monitoring, which should involve collaboration between drug manufacturers and PCCs, and which could utilise the computerised case file. Currently, we are catching up with collation of case data for existing drugs, and we are also seeking, with the assistance of the Association of the British Pharmaceutical Industry (ABPI), to establish a database on new products as they enter large scale clinical trials, especially if the products concerned are considered prime subjects for self-poisoning. Overdosage with trial drugs has occurred before, for example, with mexiletine [12] whilst overdosage with the new hypnotics, anxiolytics and antidepressants is usually almost simultaneous with their release if it has not already been reported. To date, we have a small number of files on drugs undergoing U.K. trials. May I take this opportunity to ask other manufacturers to provide us with similar data on their products?

Conclusions

1. LD50 test results are of little value for the prediction of acute drug toxicity in man.
2. Acute animal studies are of use if they:
    a) Give some approximate indication of the order of acute toxicity.
    b) Study the toxic effects rather than simply record death.
3. Maximum use should be made of the information gathered in the diagnosis and management of acute drug poisoning in man.

References

1. British Toxicology Society (1984) A new approach to the classification of substances and preparations on the basis of their acute toxicity. Human Toxicol 3, 85–92
2. Court H, Volans GN (1984) Poisoning after overdose with nonsteroidal anti-inflammatory drugs. Adv Drug React Ac Pois Rev 3, 1–21

3. Court H, Streete P and Volans GN (1983) Acute poisoning with ibuprofen. Human Toxicol 2, 381–384
4. Crome P (1982) Antidepressant overdosage. Drugs, 23, 431–461
5. Edwards JN, Volans GN and Wiseman HM (1984) Poisons Informations Proceedings: The Development of a Computer Database for Case Records. In: Current Perspectives in Health Computing. (Ed. Kostrewski B). Cambridge Univ Press, Cambridge, pp 141–154
6. Edwards JN, Wiseman HM and Volans GN (1984) Computer storage and retrieval of human case data on acute poisoning. (Abstract) XIth Int Cong Eur Assoc Poison Control Centres, Stockholm
7. Forshell GP (1975) The distribution and excretion of (^{3}H, ^{14}C) Lofepramine in the rat. Xenobiotica, 5, 73–82
8. Forshell GP (1977) The absorption, excretion and plasma protein binding of Lofepramine in the rat, dog and man. Xenobiotica, 7, 153–164
9. Goulding R and Volans GN (1980) Poisons Information Services. In: Monitoring for Drug Safety. (Ed Inman, WHW) MTP Press, London, pp 367–377
10. Heath A (1984) Suicidal overdoses of antidepressants, with special reference to Lofepramine. International Medicine (Supplement Number 10), 27–30
11. Henry JA and Volans GN (1984) ABC of Poisoning – Analgesic Poisoning: I – salicylates. Br med J 2, 820–822
12. Jequier P, Jones R and Mackintosh A (1976) Fatal mexiletine overdose. Lancet, I, 429
13. Lindbom LO and Forsberg T (1981) Cardiovascular effects of Zimelidine and other antidepressants in conscious rats. Acta Psych Scand 63 (Suppl 290) 380–384
14. Merck E (1983) Promotional literature for GAMANIL.
15. National Poison Information Service Monitoring Group (1981) Analgesic Poisoning: A Multi-centre, Prospective Survey. Human Toxicol 1, 7–23
16. Roche L (1979) Toxicologie Clinique Centre Anti-Poisons: Toxicovigilance. Bull Med Leg Toxicol 22, No 5, 570–581
17. Runkel R, Chaplin MD, Sevelius H, Ortega E and Segre E (1976) Pharmacokinetics of naproxen overdosage. Clin Pharmacol Therap 20, 269–277
18. Volans GN (1984) The Role of Poison Control Centres (PCCs) in Epidemiological Studies. Paper presented at a meeting in Rio de Janeiro in July 1984 entitled "Toxicovigilance and Public Health: The Role of Poison Control Centres"
19. Volans GN (1984) The Role of Poison Control Centres in Prevention of Poisoning Incidents and in Education. Paper presented at a meeting in Rio de Janeiro in July 1984 entitled "Toxicovigilance and Public Health: The Role of Poison Control Centres"
20. Widdop B (1982) Application of toxicological analyses in the diagnosis and management of poisoning. XIth International Congress of Clinical Chemistry. W de Gruyter and Co Berlin and New York, pp 911–919
21. Wiseman HM, Guest K and Volans GN (1984) Drug packaging and childhood poisoning. (Abstract) XIth Int Cong Eur Assoc Poison Control Centres, Stockholm.

Discussion following Dr. Oliver and Dr. Volans

Classification of chemicals by overt toxicity is important in proposing rules and safety precautions for the handling and use of chemicals. Any system of classification may suffer from the rigidity of the boundaries separating the different classes. A difference of 1 mg/kg in acute toxicity may put a substance into a different group with major consequences for its ease of use in commerce. The LD50 appears to be an attractive criterion for classification, because it depends on the most definite of all biological responses, life or death. This means that it is very easy for regulatory agencies and for industry to use it. It is very difficult to replace such a simple concept. Many other data can be obtained from acute toxicity study, but at the present time it is not easy to find another classification system.

DR. OLIVER

The current guidelines proposed by OECD do stipulate that one must make extra observations, for example, with regard to symptomatology. Additional clinical signs which are important, for example, methemoglobinemia or cyanosis must be reported. If you decide that they are the most important features, then you must actually classify your compound according to the appearance of that clinical sign. This may be more accurate than to use the lethal dose as the assessment point. However, it must be recognised that it would be very difficult to introduce a general classification system on this basis.

The toxicologist has an important role in trying to classify compounds in this way. A regulatory agency has an equally important role in assessing whether the classification is suitable or not.

DR. MORGENROTH

The particular issue about the differences between different types of limit doses is on an OECD agenda for discussion. OECD test guidelines on acute toxicity are being reviewed at present by the OECD Updating Panel.

The proposals for changes in OECD guidance were welcomed.

DR. VOLANS

Information about the clinical signs and course of acute intoxication gained from animal studies has been of limited value in guiding clinicians in how to diagnose and deal with acute poisoning in man. Similarly, on the few occasions when they have been undertaken, trials of different treatments of acute poisoning in animals have generally been more valuable in devising therapies than an understanding of kinetics, protein binding etc.

There have been few critical attempts to compare the features of acute intoxication in man and animals. The availability of comprehensive databases should make it possible to do such analyses using the many thousands of reports and queries received each year by National Poisons Centres. The British National Poisons Centre has 40,000 enquiries a year, half of which are related to medicines, about 2,500 to industrial chemicals and about 1,500 to agro-chemicals. The data on human experience are limited but they are readily available for evaluation.

Acute Toxicology Viewed from the Pharmaceutical Industry

M. Schach von Wittenau

Toxicology as a science is evolving no less rapidly than other fields of biology. The tools available to investigators are varied and powerful, and forever are increasing in number and sophistication. Although toxicologists frequently have a separate organizational identity, and their orientation is different from that of pharmacologists, they obviously are part of the research community which investigates the interaction of chemicals with living organisms. While they are as eager as their fellow scientists in other disciplines to use the best available method for obtaining knowledge, they are shackled by the task assigned to most of them, that is safety assessment of chemicals. The toxicologist practising his profession to evaluate whether or not a chemical is "safe" under the anticipated conditions of use, labors in the public arena and must do what societal consensus prescribes. He is not an unencumbered scientist, free to do what his judgement indicates, but is expected to conform to procedures dictated by society. While he can and must seize the initiative to bring about changes, he cannot unilaterally implement these but has to wait for consensus to be achieved. As his activities must meet with approval literally around the world, he serves many masters who are inclined to feel that more is better.

Toxicology and safety assessment are not identical activities, although the latter is not possible without the former. The safety assessment of drugs draws on knowledge obtained from *in vitro* studies, animal experiments, and clinical observations. Each of these three methods is capable of providing unique information, but the relative contribution each field can make changes with the developing state of the art, and also differs from case to case. As the available tools become more sophisticated and complex, critical re-examinations of current practices are indicated to ascertain that studies are designed appropriately and still serve the functions once assigned to them.

The final judgement as to the safety of pharmaceuticals is rendered by the physician. In large measure, he will base his opinion on clinical data. The relative importance of knowledge gained from experiments with laboratory animals retrospectively may seem small, yet clinical studies could not have been initiated without them. Early in the development of a drug, the physician's decision to evaluate a new chemical in man rests entirely upon assurance provided by the toxicologist, whose contribution, however, becomes nonessential once adequate experience in man has been obtained.

Acute toxicity testing of drugs in an integral part of safety assessment. Approximately fifty years ago, when most drugs were developed for short-term use, such testing may have represented the bulk of the animal experiments conducted. At that time, the methodology became standardized and was refined to yield rather precise numbers for the median lethal dose under the conditions of the experiment. Since then the LD50 test has been considered by many as the technically correct method for evaluating the acute toxicity of drugs, despite some severe criticism pointing to the limited usefulness of the information obtained [2, 3].

As questions regarding the potential health hazard to man shifted in focus towards consequences of long-term exposure, methodologies utilizing laboratory animals became more elaborate. Today, drugs are administered for weeks, months and years to mimic potential human use. Although acute toxicology studies were continued in the classical LD50 format, they represented a decreasing share of all toxicology experiments and LD50 values dwindled in importance. The almost universal perception that the rigorous determination of the LD50 was the only acceptable format for acute studies, a view which was reinforced by practically all guidelines which addressed acute toxicology assessments, provides the reason for the endurance into very recent times of the LD50 test as a routine procedure in drug safety evaluation.

Early in 1982, the Drug Safety Subsection of the US Pharmaceutical Manufacturers Association (PMA) examined the then current practices of acute toxicology testing, the reason for the procedures followed, and the utility of the data obtained. As stated earlier, in accord with numerous guidelines and textbook procedures, the LD50 format was applied. It was widely believed that this was the thing to do, and that such experiments were expected by regulatory agencies. The perception regarding this latter point had been reinforced occasionally by requests for additional LD50 data.

It was apparent, however, that during the development of a new drug the precise LD50 number had no intrinsic value. Toxicologists designing the pivotal studies expected to yield information needed by the physician supervising initial clinical trials, usually conducted range finding experiments, which suggested maximum tolerated doses, but did not generate precise numbers of lethality. Similarly, the clinical investigator wanted to know which doses did not harm animals, and what to look for in his volunteers to detect tolerance problems as early as possible. He is interested in subtle changes caused by the multiple administration of sublethal doses to laboratory animals. Thus, the LD50 determination had become an exercise conducted to facilitate approval for marketing of a new drug and no longer served as a guide either to the toxicologist or the clinician.

As I alluded to earlier, toxicologists are not free to change procedures unilaterally. The PMA, therefore, attempted to foster the building of a consensus on this issue, and published a position paper [1] which culminated in the following three proposals:

"1. The precise determination of an LD50 value should be limited to those rare cases where it is scientifically necessary for the comparison of potencies of different batches of the same chemical, or of different chemicals of very similar structure and/or activity.
2. An effort to obtain a maximum amount of scientific information from the use of a minimum number of animals should be encouraged in acute safety studies. An approximate LD50 value and/or definition of a range for toxic doses usually represents adequate information on the acute toxicity of drugs, for which many other toxicologic data are available.

3. Drugs usually are developed for worldwide distribution. Consequently, toxicology protocols are designed to meet the regulations of the most demanding country. Efforts should be made toward achieving agreement from all regulatory agencies that for drugs a precise LD50 determination is not necessary."

In the US, the response generally was very encouraging. In November 1983, the FDA sponsored a symposium which served to clarify the position of various government agencies. FDA does not now, and in fact maintained never to have explicitly required as part of a New Drug Application the determination of an exact LD50 value. To make sure that such requirement is not implied, FDA is now removing from its statements any ambiguity which could be understood as indicating that such data are expected to be submitted to them. PMA members sincerely hope that a worldwide consensus can be reached on this point.

In the meantime, and anticipating a consensus, PMA members are attempting to obtain the desirable acute toxicity information with as little animal use as possible. Basically, three approaches are being followed. A limit test, which established toleration of a relatively high dose may in some instances demonstrate adequate acute safety of a drug, and permit starting multiple dose studies. Alternatively, a modification of the classical procedure assigns fewer animals to each dose group; generally, 2–5 rodents may be used. In addition, the minimum number of dosage groups feasible for indicating the lethal range are employed. Sparing of animals also may be possible by not fully duplicating the experiment in both sexes. Another approach is the so-called "up-down method". In this, drug is administered to one animal at a dose thought to be close to the true LD50. The animal is observed for the usual 7 or 14 days, but if it has survived for one day, another animal is then given a higher dose, and it too is similarly observed. On the next day, a third animal receives either a higher or a lower dose, depending upon the fate of the second animal. Thus, by adjusting each dose up or down for each successive animal, depending upon the survival of its predecessor, a median lethal dose can be estimated as long as death is not delayed beyond one day.

It is hoped that the resulting data obtained by any of these three or any other similarly appropriate method which may emerge, will be found acceptable. At this point, I am not aware of any problem having arisen. In the debate about substitutes for the classical LD50 procedures, sight must not be lost of the fact that the only legitimate needs that must be met are those of the clinical investigator. Guiding dosage selection for multiple dose toxicology experiments often may become the main function of acute studies. The temptation should be resisted to mandate directly by regulation, or implicitly by guideline a rigid procedure. As far as the PMA is concerned, it does not intend at this time to recommend one method over others so that investigators are free to select in each instance the most appropriate approach.

References

1. LeBeau JE (1983) Regul Toxicol Pharmacol 3: 71–74
2. Sperling F (1976) Advances in modern Toxicology 1/1, pp 177–191
3. Zbinden G, Flury-Roversi M (1981) Arch Toxicol 47: 77–99

Discussion

To obtain the concerted view of the US Pharmaceutical Industry on a topic is difficult, even when the issues are as clear as the relative value and position of the LD50 and acute toxicity test. Individual toxicologists in particular companies may differ over points of detail. They would all support the consensus opinion presented here.

It is unfortunate that in many instances the industrial need for rapid progress requires scientists to fulfill regulatory requirements in a check-list fashion rather than critically appraising the real scientific need for various types of safety data. In this context it was the view of the PMA that for most purpose the flexible range-finding type of study would provide all the worthwhile information sought in an acute toxicity test, i.e. limited experiments in which a small range of doses was administered for set periods, and in which sufficient observations were made to indicate the target organs for toxicity.

A question was asked about which countries still required the formal LD50 test in marketing applications for new pharmaceutical agents?

It was pointed out that the delays in regulatory systems meant that it would take several years before any loosening of official requirements could work through to the production of appropriately diminished data by the industry.

In Vitro Models for Acute Toxicity Testing

J. M. Frazier

The basic problem faced by the pharmaceutical industry is to provide efficacious products which are safe for use by the intended consumer. Literally hundreds of new products and formulations are developed each year which must be evaluated for all aspects of potential toxicity. The need for simple, rapid and reliable test methods is obvious. The potential of *in vitro* tests to meet these needs is equally obvious. The advantages of *in vitro* tests over conventional whole animal tests include significant reductions in cost, time and physical resources. In addition, *in vitro* tests have the advantage of addressing the concerns of animal welfare advocates by reducing and/or eliminating the utilization of live animals in toxicity tests.

The various classes of toxicological responses for which a new product must undergo testing are listed in Table 1. For all of these toxicological classes it is important to distinguish between acute and chronic time scales. The terms acute and chronic refer to both the exposure and the duration of the response. Thus, it is possible to refer to an acute exposure (a single dose or several doses over a limited period of time – usually less than 1 week) and a chronic response (observing the effects over periods of months up to the life time of the animal). Other possible combinations of exposure and response time scales can also be investigated. Here we are concerned with *in vitro* approaches to acute toxicity testing, i.e. alternatives to whole animal studies involving a single exposure and responses occuring in the acute phase – up to two weeks. In general, the current whole animal tests in this category are designed to give two pieces of information:
1. definition of potential target organs, and
2. a relative index of toxicity – LD50/ED50.

As a secondary benefit of such studies, knowledge concerning the symptoms and time course of the toxic response is obtained. The ultimate question is, can *in vitro* toxicity tests be designed to replace this type of whole animal testing. Clearly, a single *in vitro* test will never be sufficient to replace the complicated systemic interactions which

Table 1. Various classes of toxicity testing which new products must undergo

---
Inflammation and Irritation
Genotoxicity – Mutagenicity/Carcinogenicity
Teratogenicity
General/Organ Specific Cytotoxicity

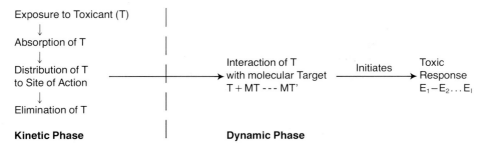

Fig. 1. The Toxicological Process

influence the intact animal experiment. However, it is conceivable that in the long run a battery of *in vitro* tests could serve this function with greater accuracy and precision due to the greater experimental control possible with *in vitro* tests.

In order to get a better perspective of the question at hand, let us stand back for a moment and review the components of the fundamental toxicological process occuring *in vivo*. Figure 1 gives a schematic diagram of what is called the Toxicological Process. This conceptualization is based on the fundamental principal that ultimate toxicity is a consequence of the molecular interaction of the active agent with a molecular target at the cellular level, where the molecular target can be an enzyme, DNA, membrane phospholipid, structural protein, etc. The overall toxicological process can be divided into two components:
1. the kinetic phase, and
2. the dynamic phase.

The kinetic phase involves all those processes which determine the relationship between exposure to a substance and the concentration of the potentially active form of that agent at the target cell. Potentially active form means either the ultimate active chemical species or a species which can be converted to the ultimate active form within the target cell.

Some of the factors which will have a significant influence on this phase are summarized in Table 2. The second phase of the overall process, the dynamic phase, is basically the cellular response to the agent. Whether or not toxicity occurs depends on the combination of processes listed in Table 2. If the agent, as presented to the cell, is not the ultimate toxic form, then cytotoxicity will require activation in the target cell.

Table 2. Factors which influence the *in vivo* toxicity of a chemical agent

I. Kinetic Phase	II. Dynamic Phase
a) Lipid solubility	a) Nature of interaction at molecular target
b) Membrane transport	b) Intracellular metabolism
c) Macromolecular binding	c) Repair mechanisms
d) Metabolism	d) Compensation mechanisms
	e) Detoxification mechanisms
	f) Physiological state

Lack of enzyme systems required to activate the agent will prevent cytotoxicity in this particular cell type. The nature of the interaction between the agent and its molecular target will be important since a reversible molecular interaction will allow rapid recovery of function when the agent is removed. Irreversible interaction will mean that a permanent alteration will persist even when the agent is dispersed.

The type of interaction will have a significant influence on the relationship between level/duration of cellular exposure to the agent and the time course of toxicological events. The ultimate cellular damage caused by the agent will be controlled by the balance between the damage produced and the ability of the cell to repair and compensate for the damage and/or detoxify the agent. Finally, the susceptibility to toxic effects can depend on the physiological state of the cell. For example, hormonal effects can alter the biochemical status of the cell, either increasing or decreasing the likelihood of a toxic result. In order to completely evaluate the acute toxicity potential of a new agent or formulation it will be necessary to develop a battery of *in vitro* measurements and tests to obtain sufficient information to predict all aspects of *in vivo* behavior.

Getting back to the focus of this symposium, acute toxicity, we will discuss *in vitro* alternatives relating to general/organ specific acute cytotoxicity. When considering the development of a new *in vitro* test it is necessary to define the goal of such a test. We begin by asking the question: What information was derived from the *in vivo* test which the *in vitro* test is to replace? For acute toxicity testing, we are particularly concerned with defining target organs and establishing some relative ranking of the toxic potential of an agent. The second question then becomes: How well does the *in vivo* test perform (false positives / false negatives / relative ranking of toxicity)? And thirdly does the test attain societal goals? These not only include the health and welfare of human beings but also the conservation and humane treatment of animal resources. Based on these considerations it may be concluded that *in vitro* testing approaches may better serve society.

In order to develop new approaches to toxicity tests, one of two possible events must occur. Either there must be the development of new knowledge at the fundamental, scientific level or there must be new technological developments. At the scientific level, what is required is the investigation of new *in vitro* systems and the evaluation of new biochemical/physiological/morphological endpoints as potential indices of toxicity. As discussed below, this is a major objective of The Johns Hopkins Center for Alternatives to Animal Testing. On the technological side, developments in maintaining specific, differentiated cell types in defined media are necessary as well as the development of new and sophisticated measurement techniques for determining toxicity endpoints. Particularly important are new techniques to utilize human cell cultures. New developments along these lines open new avenues for *in vitro* test development.

Having first established the need for new *in vitro* toxicity tests to replace currently utilized acute toxicity tests, and second the scientific and technological basis for new tests, it is necessary to carry out a validation program. The critical question is: Does the new *in vitro* test provide as good or better data than the *in vivo* test which it is to replace? For acute toxicity testing it is apparent that a battery of *in vitro* tests will be required to establish beyond a reasonable doubt the potential organ specificity and

Table 3. The goals of the Center for Alternatives to Animal Testing

1. to encourage fundamental research needed for the development of *in vitro* test procedures or other non-whole-animal test procedures which examine the toxicity of chemical compositions
2. to develop and validate methodology that will provide alternative approaches to live animal studies for the evaluation of safety
3. to encourage and promote the acceptance of applicable methods of non-whole-animal safety testing
4. to disseminate the information developed to all audiences so that appropriate change in scientific procedures and policies can occur

relative toxicity of new agents. These new tests must provide an accurate profile of potential toxicity if the use of whole animal testing is to be completely eliminated. In the short run, *in vitro* tests based on animal cell cultures can significantly reduce the number of animals utilized in testing programs. In the long term a spectrum of toxicity tests using human cells will eliminate both the traditional problem of species extrapolation and the need for whole animal testing.

Switching gears again, we will look at the role of The Johns Hopkins Center for Alternatives to Animal Testing in this whole process. The Center was established in 1981 through grants from the Cosmetic, Toiletry and Fragrance Association, Inc. and the Bristol Myers Company. The objectives of the Center are listed in Table 3. To date the major activity of the Center is to establish both intramural and extramural research programs. In the past year the Center has funded 22 research projects – 10 intramural /12 extramural. These projects have been classified into three catagories, Table 4. Research in these program areas is directed towards establishing new fundamental knowledge about potential toxicity indices in new test systems. Following identification of potential test systems the program encourages the establishment of a standard test protocol which can then be put through a validation process.

Table 4. CAAT research catagories

1. Irritation and Inflammation
2. Cytotoxicity – Acute Toxicity
3. Organ Specific Effects

The first objective of the scientific program is to develop alternatives to the use of live animals for skin, eye and mucous membrane irritation testing. The individual projects are aimed at supplying the component pieces of the irritant and/or inflammatory response. Each of the programs, intramurally (at present) and extramurally during the coming years, will be using similar test compounds in each of their systems. This coordination should lead to reliable, less expensive and acceptable (to government and societal groups) *in vitro* toxicological testing methods. Specific projects in this component of the scientific program include:

a) A study of the release of prostaglandins by rat vaginal slices in primary culture as an indication of tissue irritation produced by test compounds (Norman H. Dubin, The Johns Hopkins School of Medicine, Baltimore, MD).
b) A study of wound healing in human corneal cells grown *in vitro*. An eye irritation test based on human corneal cultures would be quicker, cheaper and more accu-

rate than the Draize eye test (Marcia M. Jublatt and Arthur H. Neufeld, Eye Research Institute, Boston, MA).

c) A study of the release of plasminogen activator, a protein associated with eye injury, by cultured rabbit corneal cells, as a potential index of eye irritation (Kwan Y. Chan, University of Washington School of Medicine, Seattle, WA).

d) A study of prostaglandin metabolism in endothelial cells cultured from human umbilical cord as an index of irritation (David Newcombe, The Johns Hopkins School of Hygiene and Public Health, Baltimore, MD).

e) A study of the release of lymphokines by primary cultures of rabbit and human skin to evaluate dermal irritation (Arthur M. Dannenberg, Jr., The Johns Hopkins School of Hygiene and Public Health, Baltimore, MD).

f) A study of the release of lysosomal enzymes by fibroblasts *in vitro* as an index of chemical damage to interstitial tissues (Sharon S. Krag, The Johns Hopkins School of Hygiene and Public Health, Baltimore, MD).

g) A study of the transport of chemicals across an artificial skin (filter paper impregnated with lipids) as a model system to replace whole animal test to determine dermal absorption of cosmetics and drugs (Richard H. Guy, University of California School of Medicine, San Francisco, CA).

h) A study of the photoxocity of chemicals in human peripheral blood monocytes as a replacement for whole animal phototoxicity testing (John A. Parrish, Harvard Medical School and Massachusetts General Hospital, Boston, MA).

i) The development of an *in vitro* epithelial-connective tissue matrix barrier model system to investigate the effects of chemicals on barrier function (Philip H. Sannes, The Johns Hopkins University School of Hygiene and Public Health Baltimore, MD).

j) The development of an *in vitro* membrane culture to investigate the effect of chemical agents on tight junction integrity and membrane fluidity (Michael A. Edidin, The Johns Hopkins School of Arts and Sciences, Baltimore, MD).

A second objective of the scientific program is to develop testing procedures that will evaluate cytotoxicity or acute toxicity. At the present time, liver cells are the major cell type employed in these studies. Liver cells were selected since they contain the whole spectrum of xenobiotic metabolizing enzymes. However, mechanisms uncovered in these cells will translate to other cell types. All five projects using liver cells involve measurement of changes in cell function after exposure to putative toxins. These *in vitro*, or test tube, methods not only will decrease the number of animals used in toxicity testing but also provide a deeper understanding of the functional role of the liver, a key player in the body's response to toxins. The work with cultured liver cells will lead to new test protocols that can be utilized in acute toxicity testing. The following projects are currently supported by the Center:

a) A study of the effect of chemical toxins on cytochrome P450 metabolism of drugs and other metabolic functions of rat hepatocytes. These endpoints are potential indices of cytotoxicity (Genvieve Krack, Catholic University of Louvain, School of Pharmacy, Brussels).

b) A study of the influence of chemical agents on the proliferation of peroxisomes (intracellular vesicles containing enzymes important for biochemical reactions) in primary cultures of rat hepatocytes (Timothy J. B. Gray, British Industrial Research Association, Carshalton, England).

c) A study of the role of calcium in the cytotoxic process in order to understand the mechanism of action of hepatotoxins (Daniel Acosta, Jr. and Elsie M. Sorensen, The University of Texas at Austin, College of Pharmacy, Austin, Texas).
d) A study of the synthesis and secretion of acute reactive proteins by mouse hepatocytes in response to exposure to toxic agents (David J. Thomas, The Johns Hopkins University, John F. Kennedy Institute, Baltimore, MD).
e) A study of the induction of specific cellular proteins in rat hepatocytes as a potential index of cytotoxic responses (John M. Frazier, The Johns Hopkins School of Hygiene and Public Health, Baltimore, MD).

A third objective of the Center's scientific program is organ specific toxicity. These projects are aimed at developing methods to assess the acute and chronic effects of chemicals on specific organ systems and to provide *in vitro* methodology that will become standard and provide acceptable protocols in areas where standards have not yet been developed (e.g. teratology). Current research activities in the programatic area include:

a) Studies of synchronously beating embryonic heart cells in culture to investigate cardiac toxins (David J. Miletick, Michael Reese Hospital and Medical Center, Chicago, IL).
b) A study of the induction of phospholipidosis in cultured lung macrophages as an index of cellular dysfunction (Mark J. Reasor, West Virginia University Medical Center, Morgantown, West Virginia).
c) A study of the utilization of cultured renal medullary cells for evaluating nephrotoxic agents (Peter H. Bach, Robens Institute of Industrial and Environmental Health and Safety, University of Surrey, England).
d) A study of the use of isolated renal tubules from rabbits for the detection and investigation of nephrotoxins (A. Jay Gandolfi, The University of Arizona, Tucson, AZ).
e) A study of the potential use of a hybrid cell line for the evaluation of neuronal toxicity (Harvey S. Singer, The Johns Hopkins School of Medicine, Baltimore, MD).
f) The development of a teratogen test based on the induction of heat shock proteins in cells cultured from human amniotic fluid (Nicole Bournias-Vardiabasis, City of Hope National Medical Center, CA).

Many of the research projects supported by the Center will lead to new, *in vitro*, methods of product safety testing. Others are providing the scientific framework necessary for further research and development and will permit the Center to fulfill its objectives to develop a wide range of *in vitro* procedures as substitutes for routine toxicological tests. Tests based on mechanistic knowledge will ensure validity and acceptability.

In conclusion it can be reiterated that there are strong societal pressures to develop alternative approaches to acute toxicity testing. The Johns Hopkins Center for Alternatives to Animal Testing, along with other internationally recognized organizations, is playing a major role in providing the necessary scientific basis for development of new approaches. In the short run it is clear that *in vitro* techniques are not sufficiently developed to replace whole animal research. However, a toxicologic profile for new chemical agents based on a battery of *in vitro* tests will provide an alternative approach to acute toxicity testing. In the near future the goal is to reduce the use of whole animals in acute toxicity testing requirements to a minimum. Ultimately, when knowledge of the fundamental principles of toxicology has significantly developed, it will be possible to eliminate the use of live animals in toxicological testing.

Discussion following Dr. Schach von Wittenau and Prof. Frazier

DR. FRAZIER

Mutual misunderstanding by regulatory agencies and industry of each other's opinions has lead to confusion about just what data scientists and government officials may consider appropriate for safety evaluation purposes. Acute studies just to provide an indication of target organs and to rank toxicity represented information that might more easily be obtained from "alternative" methods than the more basic mechanistic information required for scientific studies.

Responsible toxicologists are inevitably reluctant to abandon long established techniques that have been of definite value until they are convinced that a new "alternative" method will give results that are just as valuable and of demonstrated validity. The inherent restriction of non-animal systems to a narrow range of possible responses means that toxicologists will have to choose those systems most likely to demonstrate effects that *a priori* knowledge suggests are likely to occur. In every discussion about alternatives it is essential to be clear about what sort of effect is to be used as the end point and how useful it will be in guiding decisions about the likely safety of the substances tested.

II. Current Regulatory View on Acute Toxicity Testing

DR. GRIFFIN (Chairman)

I am very pleased to have been invited to share this session on the current regulatory review of acute toxicity testing. In 1981, Professor Zbinden wrote an excellent paper on the significance of the LD50 test for toxicological evaluation of chemical substances. His pre-publication copy and my reply were published in the Archives of Toxicology in 1981. The correspondence was picked up by the antivivisectionist movement, which, through their publication "The Animal Defender", suggested that their readers send me a letter protesting about the use of the LD50 test, proposing what measures might be taken to restrict the use of the test and advancing alternative methods. The suggestions for alternatives grieve me most. Of the 287 letters received, 20 suggested alternatives. The alternatives ranged from the use of criminals through to use of the irretrievably mentally ill. Clearly, the level of emotion applied to the use of this test has caused a loss of a sense of reality.

At that time the EC Directives 65/65 and 75/318 required an LD50 test with 95% fiducial limits. The guidelines proposed that acute toxicity tests should be conducted in such a way as to reveal acute toxicity and the mode of death. This test guideline has now been reviewed and the guideline has been substantially improved as a result of the work of Professor Bass.

EEC/CPMP

R. Bass

Introduction

In the European Community, drug registration and, therefore, the laws and regulations governing investigations into the safety of new drugs and instructions and requirements for acute toxicity testing are embedded within a framework of European regulations and national drug laws. This framework has three levels:
1. general requirements
2. Notes for Guidance and
3. national laws and regulations.

Since the policy of the Federal Health Office of the Federal Republic of Germany and subsequently of the Committee for Proprietary Medicinal Products (CPMP) of the EC towards acute toxicity testing has recently changed quite drastically, special attention will be given to regulation in this area.

Following a historical overview, the intentions and content of the proposed Notes for Guidance on Single Dose Toxicity will be described and discussed with special attention to LD50 and the value of data from acute toxicity testing.

Levels of Regulation

The rules and regulations are on three levels.

Level 1 A general text presented in the form of an EC Council Directive recommends the general types of studies to be performed and data required for granting marketing authorizations of proprietary medicinal products. Council Directive 75/318/EEC, as amended, describes analytical, pharmacotoxicological and clinical testing standards and protocols.

Level 2 The Safety Working Party of the CPMP has written Notes for Guidance which describe some areas of toxicological testing in more detail. They practically tell pharmaceutical manufacturers how they should deal with the Council Directive in order to obtain marketing authorization for a new drug in EC member states.

The Notes for Guidance were prepared by the CPMP in consultation with manufacturers' associations at both the national and at the EC levels. They were then proposed to the Council which, in turn, in its Recommendation 83/571/ECC, recommended that, for the conduct of tests and for the presentation of results, the principles set out and the methodology described in the Notes for Guidance be followed both by those applying for authorizations to place proprietary medicinal products on the market and those who examine and evaluate such applications.

Level 3 National laws and regulations have had to be changed to accord with these European regulations. In Germany, this is done in accordance with Section 26 of the Drug Act. Such rules, which combine the EC requirements with existing national requirements, are now being prepared in the Federal Republic of Germany and other EC member states.

As of today, the following Notes for Guidance have been annexed to Council Recommendation 85/371/EEC:

Annex I   Repeated dose toxicity

Annex II Reproduction studies

Annex III Carcinogenic potential

Annex IV Pharmacokinetics and metabolic studies in the safety evaluation of new drugs in animals

Annex V   Fixed combination products

As the Annex on Fixed Combination Products has no major impact on the safety aspect of testing, it will not be discussed in this paper. The texts of these Guidelines were published in the Official Journal of the European Community (1983).

Notes for Guidance have also been prepared for mutagenicity testing but have not yet been passed by the council. Since they will appear in European drug regulation for the first time, they have still to be implemented at the national level. Other relevant areas have not yet been covered.

Acute Toxicity Testing

Acute toxicity testing usually comes first. Why has it not yet been included? The answer to this question sounds almost like a fairy tale: Once upon a time there was a Council Directive 75/318/EEC which, in Chapter 1, B. 1 of Part 2 of the Annex, contained requirements for the performance of single dose (acute) toxicity testing which was supplemented by a proposal for a Note for Guidance on the same subject. This has long since disappeared. Its replacements were drafted by the Safety Working Party and accepted by both the CPMP and the pharmaceutical manufacturers' associations, but have not yet been passed by the Council. As we all know, this is a time-consuming, weary process. Nevertheless, we assume that the Notes will be passed in the near future. Therefore, we have to take them into consideration and act according to their contents.

Why were the proposed rules for single dose toxicity testing replaced? The old proposal was based on quite precise information on LD50's. This proposal called for and led to accumulation of data which were meant to allow a precise categorization of drugs into classes like those often used for chemicals, i.e. very toxic up to 25 mg/kg LD50 values, toxic from 25–200 mg/kg and "harmful" from 200 to 2000 mg/kg. Such schemes are dealt with in this volume by Morgenroth. The few reasons for obtaining precise information on statistically significant numbers on lethal doses are well known.

Such point estimations have their intrinsic problems. They can, depending on the substance being studied, experimental set-up and personal ability of the performer, be manipulated at ease. From collaborative studies we know that, when testing the same substance in different laboratories, both guidance and good will are necessary to reach results which are at least within the same wide range. From data supplied to our office, it is clear that very often no relationship exists between lethality numbers and the mechanism of toxic action. Limited observation periods following the single administration of the drug make the numbers even more meaningless. Since in our office one person is responsible for looking at acute and chronic toxicity (this job is not split among specialists for each test system), we soon became aware of deviations between results from the various toxicity tests and LD50 values. One third of the LD50 measured were not in a range compatible with results from chronic studies; they were either too low or too high. This was clearly not only the result of false or imprecise LD50 studies, but also misuse. These factors led to an uneasiness about using precise LD50 numbers for evaluating the toxic potential of drugs.

As our attitude changed, we began looking for better methods of evaluating acute toxicity. Since much work has been carried out in this area, the scientific methods and the technical means for an alternative approach, especially approaches to the search for changes in the function of organs and organ systems, were easily found. These methods require investigations at the level of the whole body – the whole animal. Although some features of reversibility or irreversibility, late onset of toxicity and so on can be detected by using either non-whole animal systems – and this can reach down to the molecular level – or by using LD50 type experiments, neither style seems adequate to draw out all the information that can be obtained from the typical whole-animal acute toxicity study. The details of how to obtain further information on the profile of acute toxicity in practice have already been described (see Appendix) and will not be discussed here.

How can the data obtained from these studies be used? The purpose of acute toxicity studies is to gain information on the effects of acute overdose and poisoning. This information is useful for the following pre-clinical and clinical studies. This information is required relatively early during drug development, but its importance dwindles by the time of registration. However useful and important this information was for the development of the drug, the proposition that studies yielding LD50s with high precision have to be reported at the time of registration must be refuted. If such studies are not needed early in the development of a drug, then they are equally useless later for regulatory purposes. Therefore, companies must change their practice of redoing precisely those LD50 studies which were performed earlier as acute toxicity tests and judged by toxicologists and clinicians to be sufficient to allow further development. Avoidance of such duplication will save a lot of animals. Furthermore, when planning and performing acute toxicity studies, we must not forget that sometimes relevant information is already available, e.g. from pharmacological studies and from safety pharmacology investigations. This should influence the kind and extent of acute toxicity testing and, therefore, lead to the avoidance of unnecessary duplication of results and to expensive answers to irrelevant questions.

During further development of the drug, we should not forget our original acute toxicity data. Reevaluation should be made as we gain knowledge, for example, on pharmacokinetic behavior and from clinical studies. We can then possibly make much better use of results and data which were quite misunderstood earlier.

Our position on acute toxicity studies was reached by very close cooperation among scientists from academia and industry and our staff. The result, a paper on new – or as some would put it – old ways to carry out acute toxicity testing, was published in 1982 as a combined statement by outstanding members of academia and industry together with our experts (1). The BGA immediately officially endorsed our proposal and promised to accept such studies for the safety evaluation of drugs (3).

Within the EC, the CPMP's Safety Working Party, headed by Dr. Griffin, took up our proposals and worked very hard to gain agreement on them within the EC. They were discussed with manufacturers in the EC and the results of these discussions were written up as a "Proposed Revision of Directive 75/318" and its "Annex, Note for Guidance on Single Dose Toxicity" dated January 11, 1984 (see Appendix).

With the expansion of the European Community to include Spain and Portugal, the number of countries and people relying on, or being recommended to, these regulations will increase considerably. In addition, we know from fruitful discussions with officials from the EFTA group that, although they are not bound by these rules, they agree with their principles on how drug safety testing should be performed. It is now clear that the regulatory agencies of the world's largest drug market, Western Europe, speak with one mind about acute toxicity and other areas of drug testing.

We are now trying to find world wide agreement. The different attitudes of different regulatory agencies act as multipliers which lead to the use of 1000 animals and more per drug for acute toxicity studies alone. Most of these animals can be saved and we can still obtain better information on both approximate lethal actions and acute toxicity.

Changes have already been introduced in the USA. It was a pity that we had to learn about them from the newspapers. After the implementation of the changes, we heard rumors from companies that, although LD50s were no longer required, they have still been requested. We were told this when we inquired about the reason for still performing LD50 studies. From companies and from published regulations we know that Japan keeps the issue open, so that they can ask for determination of the LD50 in several species, including dogs, and by several routes of administration. To me, this is a setback.

What can a regulatory agency do once it has realized uneasiness about a certain type of study? It can inaugurate and support scientific discussion and get things going on the national and international levels. Even in the seemingly easy area of acute toxicity, our job is not yet finished either nationally or internationally. Nationally, the impact on other areas of testing in our chemical world, the testing both of constituents and finished products, is only beginning to show. For the regulations necessary for the implementation of our Chemicals Act, we still have to define workable solutions and acceptable classifications which do not rely solely on mortality data. Internationally, the Committee of Experts on the Transport of Dangerous Goods in Geneva stated in December 1982 that precise data on LD50s and LC50s were necessary. As far as I know, this attitude has not yet changed. Furthermore, mutual acceptance of foreign data on toxicity has to be achieved, but settlement at the highest level demanded by some countries must be avoided. Agreement must be reached at the level giving the necessary information, not at the level of largest numbers of animals and species. Our task has been made easier by the arguments from animal protection groups. It is not our intention to hinder drug development by decreasing the number of animal experiments possible. Our intention is to increase the value of those experiments that have to be performed. If this leads to fewer animals required, then both ends meet. Acute toxicity testing is one area where this has already been achieved. When considering other areas of toxicological testing, we must avoid extremes: the fulfilment of demands for cutting the number of animals and experiments by some given percentage is bound to yield useless results. We know that completion of our task will take time and endurance and are willing to provide both.

Conclusion

In conclusion, let me say that acute toxicity is a formidable meeting ground for concerned scientists and animal protection groups. I believe that we can be proud of the state-of-the-art achieved thus far and its translation into regulations. Let us translate the state-of-the-art into other languages, too.

Appendix

Revision of Directive 75/318/EEC Part 2, Chapter 1, B. Toxicity

1. *Single Dose Toxicity*

   An acute test infers a qualitative and quantitative study of the toxic reactions which may result from a single administration of the active substance or substances contained in the proprietary medicinal product, in the proportions and (physico-chemical state) in which they are present in the actual product.

   The acute toxicity test must be carried out on two or more mammalian species of known strain unless a single species can be justified. At least two different routes of administration shall normally be used, one being identical with or similar to that proposed for use in human beings and the other ensuring systemic absorption of the substance.

   This study will cover the signs observed, including local reactions. The period during which the test animals are observed shall be fixed by the investigator as being adequate to reveal tissue or organ damage or recovery, usually for a period of fourteen days but not less than seven days, but without exposing the animals to prolonged suffering. Animals dying during the observation period should be subject to autopsy as also should all animals surviving to the end of the observation period. Histopathological examination should be considered on any organ showing macroscopic changes at autopsy. The maximum amount of information should be obtained from the animals used in the study. The single dose toxicity tests should be conducted in such a way that signs of acute toxicity are revealed and the mode of death assessed as far as reasonably possible. In suitable species a quantitative evaluation of the approximate lethal dose and information on the dose effect relationship should be obtained, but a high level of precision is not required.

Single Dose Toxicity:

Notes for Guidance concerning the application of the Annex to Directive 75/318/EEC, Part 2, Chapter I, paragraph B, point 1, with a view to the granting of a marketing authorization for a new drug

Introduction

These guidelines deal with the qualitative and quantitative study of toxic phenomena and their occurrence related to time after a single administration of the substance, or combination of substances.

These studies may give some indication of the likely effects of acute overdosage in man and may be useful for the design of toxicity studies requiring repeated dosing on the relevant animal species.

The single dose toxicity tests should be conducted in such a way that signs of acute toxicity are revealed and the mode of death determined. In suitable species a quantitative evaluation of the approximate lethal dose and information on the dose effect relationship should be made, but a high level of precision is not required.

Toxicologists should use their best judgments in designing the studies so that the maximal amount of relevant information is obtained from the smallest numbers of animals.

Product Specification

a) Drug substance

The active substance should be have the same pattern of impurities as the product to be marketed, when possible. Should the final dosage form be shown to have impurities significantly different either in quantity or quality from those in the test batch then further steps should be taken to ascertain their possible toxicity. Consideration should be given to the physical characteristics of the drug substances in relation to the route of administration, e.g. the particle size of a compound given orally.

b) Finished product

When large animals are used in the acute toxicity study, it may be possible to conduct a study with the pharmaceutical formulation intended to be marketed. This is particularly desirable when the pharmaceutical formulation is likely to lead to major changes in the bioavailability of the active ingredient(s).

c) Excipients

Where a new excipient is used for the first time it should be evaluated as a new active substance.

These studies may give some indication of the likely effects of acute overdosage in man and may be useful for the design of toxicity studies requiring repeated dosing on the relevant animal species.

In the case of active substances in combination, the study must be carried out in such a way as to check whether or not there is enhancement of toxicity or if novel toxic effects occur.

d) Products containing a combination of active substances

In the case of combination of active substances it is necessary to make a study of each active substance separately and of the combination of active substances in the same proportions as in the proposed final product in order to check whether or not there is enhancement of toxicity or if novel toxic effects occur. Deviations from this protocol should depend on documented pharmacokinetic or pharmacodynamic differences between the animal species studied and man.

e) Where degradation products occur under conditions of storage, consideration should be given to their possible toxicity and this might be best evaluated initially by an acute toxicity study.

Animals

a) Single dose toxicity tests must be conducted on at least two mammalian species known strain using equal numbers of both sexes. Rodents such as the mouse, rat and hamster are suitable for the qualitative study of toxic signs and the quantitative determination of the approximate lethal dose. If no difference in response is observed between the animals of the two sexes of the first rodent species, then only animals of one sex need be used in the other acute toxicity studies. Toxic signs should also be observed and recorded in detail for each animal used in the case of other mammals.

b) Whatever species or strain of animals are selected it is essential that the following information should be provided, age, sex, weight, origin and the time in the laboratory before test, whether or not the animals are classified as being free of specific pathogens, whether or not the animals have been vaccinated or submitted to any other procedure. Details of housing and environmental conditions should be given. Access to and the nature of the diet and the availability of water should be stated. All the above factors are known to affect the acute toxicity of substances.

Administration

a) Route of administration

In the case of rodents in general, two routes should be used and when possible should include those routes proposed for man and at least one should ensure full access of unchanged drug into the circulation. If the proposed route of administration to man is intravenous, then use of this route alone in animal testing is acceptable.

b) Conditions of administration

Details of administration of the product should be provided and include particulars of the vehicle or adjuvants used, method of preparing the suspension in the case of insoluble products, concentration of the solution used and the volume administered. The route and the method of administration should be clearly given. The formulation to be administered should be as bland and as close as possible to physiological pH and osmolality.

Special attention should be paid if the formulation is alkaline, acid or potentially corrosive. Exceeding the tolerable volume should be avoided. If the intravenous route is used the rate of infusion (ml/min.) and the pH and temperature of the solution administered should be provided.

If it is necessary to use more than one injection site for parenteral administration, this should be stated.

c) Dose levels

In all species used the number of dose levels should be such that the spectrum of toxicity is revealed. In rodents a quantitative estimate of the approximate lethality and the dose effect relationship should be obtained.

Observations

Animals should be observed at regular intervals and all signs of toxicity and the time of their first occurrence and their severity, duration and progression recorded. The time and mode of any death should be documented, any signs of toxicity should be presented separately for each animal.

Observation should usually be for 14 days, but should continue so long as signs of toxicity are apparent, e.g. progressive loss of weight or inhibition of growth.

Autopsy

All animals surviving to the end of the study and all animals dying during the period of observation should be subjected to autopsy. Any organ showing macroscopic changes (other than agonal changes) should be subjected to histopathological examination unless these changes are well documented and adequate explanation for them can be given on the basis of previous experience in the strain of animal used.

Presentation of Data

The result from which any calculations have been made should be given in detail, the methods of calculation used should be stated.

The toxic effects including assessment of morbidity should be described in each species and for each route of administration at all dose levels.

The investigator should draw all relevant conclusions from the data obtained in these studies.

Any significant deviations from these guidelines should be justified.

Discussion

In addition to the 10 countries of the EEC with the CPMP to guide regulatory testing of new medicines, the controlling authorities in other countries should all clearly state that they do not require a formal LD50 determination. If the results of such experiments are submitted, they should tell the companies responsible that the studies should not have been conducted. It was pleasing that the regulatory authorities of so many countries had managed to take this positive step towards changing requirements for this particular study. It is particularly good that countries such as Switzerland have an animal protection law, which prevents studies that are not ethical and forbids pain and hardship to the animals. Every animal test which has to be done in Switzerland must be reported to the authority and approval is required. Anyone submitting a request to conduct an LD50 study of the old formal type, with a large number of animals or with larger animals, would not get permission to conduct the study. If a classical study were required, the company would have to give a very good reason for deviating from the new standards, which are accepted by most regulatory authorities.

References

1. Baß R, Günzel P, Henschler D, König J, Lorke D, Neubert D, Schütz E, Schuppan D, Zbinden G (1982) LD50 versus acute toxicity, Arch Toxicol 51, 183–186
2. J Europ Commun (1983) L332, 1–32
3. Überla K, Schnieders B (1982) In reference to the paper by Bass et al 51: 183–186, Arch Toxicol 51, 187
4. Zbinden G (1986) this volume

A US/FDA View of Acute Toxicity Testing in the Evaluation of Pharmaceuticals

L. M. CRAWFORD

Scientists, lawyers, industry executives, and representatives of animal rights groups have devoted increasing efforts to the task of identifying, understanding, and dealing with the profound ethical and practical challenges the subject of animal testing presents in the U.S. It is likely great changes will take place in science of acute toxicity testing over the next several years.

The problem was taken so seriously in the Federal Government that the U.S. Food and Drug Administration in January 1984 formed a Steering Committee on research issues. Representatives of each Center and the Office of the Commissioner were named to the Committee. Their assignment was to address five issues by gathering information on agency-wide procedures, practices and requirements related to each issue.

The five issues phrased as questions were

1. Are FDA procedures so ordered as to obtain the maximum amount of useful scientific information while utilizing the fewest number of animals?
2. Do FDA procedures in any way indirectly stimulate the perpetuation of the LD50 test even though the agency no longer directly requires the use of this test?
3. Is FDA making the maximum use of and encouraging the continued development of reliable *in vitro* alternatives to *in vivo* methodologies?
4. Are mechanisms in place to ensure continuing compliance with the Animal Welfare Act and with the highest standards of animal care?
5. Is the historical usefulness of animal testing in human health protection, the primary mission of FDA, properly appreciated by our constituents?

All of the Centers and the Office of the Commissioner were represented on the Committee. The scientific background of the members included toxicology, pharmacology, veterinary medicine, microbiology and chemistry. Through its members, the Committee reviewed in depth each Center's procedures and practices related to inhouse research and research supported under contracts and grants. It also reviewed requirements imposed on industry for regulatory purposes.

I believe you will be interested in learning the answers given to the Commissioner in the committee's final report. First, let me restate the questions:

Are FDA procedures so ordered as to obtain the maximum amount of useful scientific information while utilizing the fewest number of animals?

It was found that our procedures are designed to get maximum data from the minimum number of animals. For intramural research involving animals, scientists are required to have protocols reviewed and approved before initiating a project. Part of that review focuses on the appropriate use of animals and the design of the protocol to derive scientifically reliable data from the minimum number of animals. In addition to involving statisticians in protocol development and requiring review, the agency makes continuing efforts to use *in vitro* and chemical methods to replace or minimize the use of animals in-house and in its requirements and recommendations to industry.

Perhaps the most significant contribution to the minimization of the use of animals results from the issuance of guidelines for conducting tests required to produce data necessary for a toxicological characterization of products which FDA regulates. Because of the wide range of products throughout the agency, an appreciable number of tests using a variety of animal species is required. Despite the progress being made in the use of alternatives, animals are still necessary for assessing the safety of new products. By using valid, scientifically accepted testing guidelines in-house and as requirements for industry, the maximum amount of useful data is obtained from the fewest number of animals. Without guidelines which recommend the numbers and kinds of tests and animals, data generated from inappropriate numbers and kinds of tests might result in the conduct of more tests and use of more animals than is absolutely necessary. Depending upon the product and proposed use, it may be adequate to determine only some and not all acute, subchronic and chronic effects; having guidelines helps in specifying requirements. Guidelines exist to define test protocols for evaluating safety of food and color additives, cosmetics, potency and safety of biologicals, human and veterinary drugs, and medical devices. Some also exist as part of research protocols.

Here are some guidelines to minimize the testing and use of animals

- The Center for Food Safety and Applied Nutrition (CFSAN) has issued "Toxicological Principles for the Safety Assessment of Direct Food Additives and Color Additives Used in Food". This document introduces a "concept of concern" which makes use of a tiered system for developing information for safety assessment. A procedure is outlined where, for purposes of deciding the extent of toxicity testing needed to determine safety, a compound is placed in one of three levels of concern. Initially, information on structure-activity relationships and exposure data or estimates is used to assign a compound to a concern level. The document also lists the testing requirements for each concern level. The fewest number of tests are required for Concern Level I and the most extensive testing is necessary for Concern Level III. Test guidelines are included. The Center for Food Safety and Applied Nutrition specifically states: "While this scheme does not preclude a petitioner from demonstrating safety by using other types of data elements, a submission using the agency's scheme should normally provide sufficient data to demonstrate safety."
- The Center for Veterinary Medicine (CVM) is proposing a document, "General Principles for Evaluating the Safety of Compounds Used in Food-producing Animals", for widespread distribution and use. This contains guidelines for

1. metabolism studies and identification of residues for toxicological testing,
2. toxicological testing,
3. threshold assessment,
4. establishing a tolerance,
5. approval of methods of analysis for residues, and
6. establishing withdrawal periods.

The sponsor is required to furnish information showing that residues in the edible products of treated animals are safe and the guidelines are intended to inform sponsors of the scientific information that provides an acceptable basis for such a determination. CVM's "Principles" document specifically states: "Sponsors may rely upon the guidelines with the assurance that they describe procedures acceptable to FDA. "They also give a sponsor the option to use other procedures but caution "the sponsor to discuss the propriety of the alternative procedures in advance ...". CVM also is proposing a document entitled "Target Animal Safety Guidelines for New Animal Drugs", which addresses guidelines for safety determination of new animal drugs in all animals for which a new drug may be intended. CVM says these guidelines should remain flexible to allow scientific discretion in design and execution of studies but recommends that the protocol be submitted before the trial begins.

- The Center for Devices and Radiological Health (CDRH), in its draft of "Contact Lens Product Guidelines", has suggested protocols for studies to provide data to fulfill requirements for toxicological testing, chemical testing, microbiological tests and for clinical studies of contact lens products. They also list some possible tests that provide alternatives to the use of animals and encourage efforts to continue the development of such tests. The guidelines have been designed to answer most preliminary questions but it is emphasized that potential applicants should consult with the Center's Division of Ophthalmic Devices before starting tests.
- The Center for Drugs and Biologics (CDB) has issued "Guidelines for Preclinical Toxicity Testing of Investigational Drugs for Human Use". These contain recommendations for the types of toxicologic studies in laboratory animals which must precede the various phases of clinical investigation of new drugs. With these guidelines, a major objective is to get the maximum amount of information with the minimum number of tests.

As you can see, efforts are being made continually to improve present test requirements and there are examples of modifications that resulted in the use of fewer animals. CVM has modified a test to determine animal drug tolerance in a way that has reduced the number of animals per test from 10 to not more than four. Over the past 10 to 12 years, CDRH has revised its guidelines for assessing potential toxicity of contact lenses and, as a result, has reduced the number of animals per test from 72 to 12. CDB has replaced animals completely with chemical tests for determining potency of some biological products.

Re-evaluating and improving tests – in the light of scientific development and increased knowledge – has been going on for several years. As a result, there have been reductions in the number of animals used in some tests, elimination of the need for animals in some tests and a formalization of research and testing guidelines. All of this has contributed to an overall effort to derive the maximum benefit from the minimum use of animals.

The second question asked

Do FDA procedures in any way indirectly stimulate the perpetuation of the LD50 test even though the agency no longer directly requires the use of this test?

There are many testing procedures required throughout the agency to characterize the toxic properties of chemicals but, in general, they do not directly or indirectly perpetuate the use of the traditional LD50 test.

At a workshop on acute studies, sponsored by FDA, on November 9, 1983, the conclusion was reached and a statement made that FDA has no regulations requiring use of the LD50 test. It also was stated that an approximation of this value is sufficient for all except a few highly toxic drugs such as some cancer chemotherapeutic agents. However, the Steering Committee found during its study that there is a Code of Federal Regulations (21 CFR Part 450) requirement that each of three antitumor antibiotics, because of their inherent toxicity, have LD50 data prior to batch release. The Committee also learned that the agency is considering eliminating this requirement. Several instances were found where references to the test still exist, even though there are no existing requirements for it. In every case, changes are being made to make the agency position clear.

The Steering Committee found that, in addition to specific references needing clarification, there may be instances where agency and industry scientists use the term "LD50" when they actually mean acute toxicity studies. The casual misuse of this term may be a contributing factor in the misunderstanding of FDA requirements. Some confusion also may result from the fact that when FDA, through its National Center for Toxicological Research (NCTR), conducts tests for other agencies these tests may involve LD50 determinations to meet legal requirements other than those of the FDA. The Centers have begun to take steps to resolve any misunderstanding in terms. In addition, most older guidelines have been or are being rewritten. Through review mechanism in place and current heightened awareness on the part of agency personnel, written requirements describing new or revised guidelines will reflect the position that use of this test should be avoided except for those rare situations where no alternative exists.

Here's how the third question was posed

Is FDA making maximum use of and encouraging the continued development of reliable *in vitro* alternatives to *in vivo* methodologies?

Every center within FDA has been involved for several years in the development and assessment of alternative approaches to reducing the use of animals in research. There are specific instances where requirements for animal tests have been eliminated or are being considered for elimination as the reliability of alternative procedures is validated. For example, cell culture systems have been shown to be equally or more sensitive than mice, guinea pigs and rabbits in tests for extraneous microbial agents that may be present in inactivated products such as poliomyelitis and rabies vaccines and for similar tests of live virus vaccines such as measles, mumps, rubella and the oral poliovirus vaccines. Appropriate changes in the current additional standards for these biological products will be made to delete the requirement for the use of animals in testing.

In addition, the use of cell cultures for testing the presence of residual live virus in inactivated poliomyelitis vaccine is being evaluated to determine if they are as reliable as monkeys. Preliminary results indicate that the cell culture systems may be more sensitive. For medical device products, approval has been given for industry to substitute a variety of chemical and cell culture tests for *in vivo* tests of material toxicity and identification and for quality control.

Pyrogen testing of drug products and biological products is changing from using rabbits to using Limulus Amebocyte Lysate (LAL) assay to determine the presence of bacterial endotoxins. Guidelines addressing this change have been proposed, and comments received on them are currently being reviewed. In fact, some manufacturers already have received approval to substitute LAL tests for the use of rabbits. Attempts are being made to develop *in vitro* methods to replace animal tests presently used for assaying foods for protein quality and vitamin D content.

Immunochemical and biochemical techniques are being substituted for animals to determine the potency and purity of some biological products. Analytical methodology such as spectrophotometry is used to assure potency of meningococcal and pneumococcal polysaccharide vaccines and chromatography is used to determine the identity and molecular configurations of new products using recombinant DNA technology. Single radial immunodiffusion procedures are used to determine the potency of influenza vaccines and also are currently being evaluated for determining the potency of rabies and inactivated poliomyelitis vaccines. The utility of enzyme-linked immunoassay and radioimmunoassay is also being evaluated as a suitable replacement for potency testing of poliomyelitis vaccines which currently requires the use of monkeys.

Research and development of a number of other alternative methods is being conducted or supported. Tissue culture, cell culture and subcellular cultures are being evaluated for the application to test for many substances such as heparin and protamine sulfate. Genetic probes, developed through advances in recombinant DNA technology, are being investigated for their application in assessing virulence and pathogenicity of food borne bacteria. Probes are now available for *Escherichia coli,* and *Yersinia enterocolitica* with probes under development for *Shigellae, Campylobacter jejuni, Clostridium perfringens, Bacillus cereus, Vibrio cholera, Salmonella* and *Clostridium botulinum.* The agency is following studies of cell culture methods using corneal epithelial stromal and endothelial cell lines and use of a protozoan species as alternatives to the use of animals for identification of ocular irritants.

For cosmetic ingredients, *in vitro* tests using ocular tissue cultures and cadaver skin in the Franz cell are now used frequently to provide information on skin sensitization and percutaneous absorption of cosmetic ingredients.

Unscheduled DNA synthesis, mammalian cell transformation, mouse lymphoma and the Ames Salmonella Reversion test are being investigated for their value in providing information on food additive and contaminant toxicity.

Scientists at the NCTR also use *in vitro* methods and procedures for a variety of research purposes. These include primary hepatocyte cultures for metabolism studies and the Chinese hamster ovary cells and the Ames test to determine mutagenic effects. Microorganisms, such as bacteria, yeasts and fungi, are being employed instead of animals to assess the toxicity of environmentally important chemicals.

Agency scientists are keeping abreast of activities outside FDA through attendance at scientific meetings and workshops, review of scientific literature, and professional interaction with other scientists in academia and industry. Some scientists serve as members of advisory panels or as primary consultants to professional societies or other organizations involved in studying the use of alternative methods such as the Society of Toxicology and the Johns Hopkins Center for Alternatives to Animal Testing.

The agency as a whole is actively keeping abreast of considering non-animal models for use in both research and testing. However, it is not likely that requirements for the use of animals will be eliminated soon. Efforts to reduce the use of animals, while still providing sufficient data to evaluate the toxicity of compounds, will continue at as great a pace as scientific developments justify.

The fourth question was a challenging one

Are mechanisms in place to ensure continuing compliance with the Animal Welfare Act and with the highest standards of animal care?

FDA's laboratory practices comply with the Animal Welfare Act as well as with other standards for humane care and use of animals. All centers have acceptable procedures, but they vary from center to center in specific details. For example, two facilities have full accreditation by the American Association for Accreditation of Laboratory Animal Care (AAALAC) and other facilities have acceptable self-assessment procedures for assuring proper animal care.

Accreditation by AAALAC is sought on a voluntary basis because it represents the highest form of approval for laboratory standards for animal care. It involves a visit and evaluation by experts in laboratory animal science who submit a detailed report to the Council on Accreditation. Accredited facilities submit annual status reports and are site-visited at least every three years. Full accreditation is accepted by the National Institute of Health as assurance that the animal facilities are evaluated in accordance with Public Health Service policy. In addition, there are procedures, other than through AAALAC accreditation, for assuring adherence to proper animal management practices also accepted by PHS as appropriate and adequate. This includes assurance by a responsible official that there has been a self-assessment and the facility

1. accepts as mandatory the "Principles for the Care and Use of Laboratory Animals",
2. is committed to implementing the recommendations contained in the "Guide for the Care and Use of Laboratory Animals", and
3. is complying with the Animal Welfare Act and all other applicable federal statutes and regulations.

Although not AAALAC accredited, the other FDA laboratories follow these PHS standards as well as FDA's Good Laboratory Practices regulations.

For example, the animal facilities serving the Office of Biologics Research and Review (OBRR) in the Center for Drugs and Biologics and the facilities of the National Center for Toxicological Research are both fully accredited by AAALAC. Both have formal procedures for informing their staffs of the policies on the care and use of animals. Among other things, NCTR and OBRR have adopted an "Animal Use Form for Experimental Protocols" and require every investigator using animals to provide a Committee on Care and Use of Animals with detailed information for evaluation of the protocol. Investigators are required to inform the committee of any changes in the protocol which may be required during the course of the project.

CVM has an Animal Welfare Committee that provides general oversight in the planning and conduct of intramural research. CVM requires that study designs be reviewed and approved before a project is initiated and that all nonclinical projects be monitored in accordance with an established quality assurance program. The staff, which includes two veterinarians certified by the American College of Laboratory Animal Medicine, is well qualified. Some staff members have received American Association of Laboratory Animal Science technician training and others have had in-house training in the proper care and handling of animals. The Center is moving toward AAALAC accreditation.

The Division of Toxicology in the Center for Food Safety and Nutrition also has a protocol review committee which reviews studies for compliance with established guidelines before commencement and the center has a quality assurance unit which monitors all the center's laboratory studies. Two veterinary medical officers on the staff are responsible for assuring proper animal care.

The Center for Devices and Radiological Health and the Office of Drug Research and Review of the Center for Drugs and Biologics both conduct relatively limited animal research and therefore monitor their work differently from the other centers. The Center for Devices and Radiological Health utilizes the AAALAC accredited animal welfare committee in the Office of Drug Research and Review to provide oversight and assistance. The Office of Drug Research and Review has no formal committee, but assures, through responsible supervisors, that studies are conducted in conformance with appropriate standards for animal care.

With regard to extramural programs, the agency requires that all institutions receiving awards abide by written PHS policy and procedures. This includes

1. having in place a program of animal care which meets federal and department standards,
2. providing through AAALAC accreditation or defined self-assessment procedures assurance of institutional conformance, and
3. maintaining an animal research committee to provide oversight of the institution's animal program, facilities and associated activities.

In summary, the FDA has procedures for assuring that its intramural and extramural programs and practices comply with high standards for animal care and welfare. By virtue of the nature of their program requirements and the amount of research or testing involving the use of animals, some centers have more formal procedures than others and more veterinary staff capabilities. The agency will continue to assure adherence to appropriate standards and will continue to improve facilities and procedures to establish and maintain superior standards throughout the organization.

The final question asked of the Steering Committee

Is the historical usefulness of animal testing in human health protection, the primary mission of FDA, properly appreciated by our constituents?

FDA practices and procedures demonstrate appropriate and humane use of animals and the agency supports the development of alternative tests. Development and evaluation of procedures to minimize the use of animals is a continual process. However, it is a fact that the use of animals has been and continues to be essential to determine the safety of products regulated by FDA. It is important that this requirement be recognized and understood along with the importance of promoting proper use of animals.

FDA uses a number of mechanisms for communicating its need to employ animals in fulfilling its responsibilities to protect public health. These include attendance and participation by agency personnel in meetings, workshops, conferences, symposia, etc., which provide opportunities to discuss FDA responsibilities, requirements and actions. In addition, FDA, through publications such as the *FDA Consumer* and *FDA Veterinarian,* reaches other segments of the public to inform them of FDA activities. The Office of Legislation and Information responds to Congressional inquiries in these areas. Through the Office of Science Coordination, FDA has been responding to public inquiries (as has the Office of Consumer Affairs) and has been interacting with the Office of Technology Assessment in their appraisal of "Alternatives to Animal Use in Testing and Experimentation".

These methods of communication primarily reach the public at large and are useful and important. Just as important, however, is the issuance of guidelines describing testing requirements and protocols. These are essential to industry and in most cases provide a rationale for the requirement.

Although these mechanisms do not focus exclusively on animal welfare, they are well established procedures for communicating with the broad range of FDA constituents. It is difficult to assess formally how successful FDA has been in creating an awareness of the essential role animals play, but results of polls over the past several years indicate a high degree of public awareness and approval of the agency's role in both human and animal health protection.

FDA will continue to place the use of animals in proper perspective. It also will continue its policy to improve the welfare of animals and to examine its requirements in an effort to reduce the numbers of animals needed.

Following its findings, the Steering Committee made these recommendations, which are worthy of note

1. Under the sponsorship of the Office of the Commissioner, a series of workshops should be conducted on the following issues:
   – Acute toxicity studies required throughout the agency.

   Regulatory and research staffs of the various centers would attend with the objective being to assure that everyone uses the same terms in dealing with industry. A second objective would be to inform staff members from each center of the requirements in other centers.

   – Use of *in vitro* alternatives by various centers.

   The focus would be to make staff members in each center aware of the way other centers utilize *in vitro* methodologies. The Committee found that a number of unique methods are under development and also that some of the basic methods are being used in different centers for different purposes.

   An exchange of information and views would strengthen the agency science base.

   – Agency and PHS practices and procedures for the care and handling of animals.

   Practices vary from center to center and agency staff members can benefit by sharing information. Staff members also should be informed of developments at NIH and in some other agencies because FDA participates with them in the animal welfare area.

2. Establish an agencywide animal welfare committee which would be interdisciplinary and function as a resource for the various centers and the commissioner. This committee would not have oversight responsibilities but would be advisory in nature.

   As you can see both the administrators and scientists are dedicated to keeping animal testing at a minimum, consonant with latest scientific policies and procedures and always bearing in mind our number one mission of safeguarding human health.

Current Regulatory View of Acute Toxicity Testing in Japan

M. Tezuka and A. Takanaka

A notification entitled "Information on the Guidelines of Toxicity Studies Required for Application for Approval to Manufacture (Import) Drugs, Part 1", hereinafter cited as "Toxicity Test Guideline", was jointly issued on 15th February, 1984 by the Director of Evaluation and Registration Division and the Director of Biologics and Antibiotics Division, Pharmaceutical Affairs Bureau, Ministry of Health and Welfare of Japan. The requirements for acute toxicity testing of drugs in the Toxicity Test Guideline will be introduced briefly to permit better understanding of the regulatory policy adopted for the evaluation of acute toxicity data in Japan.

Notification No. 118 of the Pharmaceutical Affairs Bureau, Ministry of Health and Welfare dated 15th February, 1984

To: Prefectural Governors

> Director
> Evaluation and Registration Division
> Pharmaceutical Affairs Bureau
> Ministry of Health and Welfare
>
> Director
> Biologics and Antibiotics Division
> Pharmaceutical Affairs Bureau
> Ministry of Health and Welfare

Information on the Guidelines of Toxicity Studies Required for Applications for Approval to Manufacture (Import) Drugs ... (Part 1).

Attached are the standard guidelines for acute toxicity, subacute toxicity, chronic toxicity, reproduction, mutagenicity and carcinogenicity studies required as data for application for approval to manufacture (import) drugs. The drug manufacturers (importers) should be thoroughly informed of the purport of these guidelines, which will be conducted as follows. Notification No. 529 of the Pharmaceutical Affairs Bureau, entitled "On studies of the effects of drugs on reproduction" issued on March 31, 1975 by Directors of the Evaluation and Registration Division and Biologics and Antibiotics Division of the Pharmaceutical Affairs Bureau, Ministry of Health and Welfare, shall be cancelled on February 29, 1984.

Notice

1. Studies* which are initiated on March 1, 1984 or after, and are utilized as data for submission of forms for application for approval to manufacture (import) drugs should be performed in accordance with the guidelines presented here.
2. Data which are attached to drug approval applications submitted on April 1, 1986 or after should be in accordance with these guidelines. Studies initiated or terminated before February 29, 1984 can be substituted as long as they satisfy the regulation for animal species noted in these guidelines in principle.

Guidelines for Toxicity Studies of Drugs

The following guidelines are intended to indicate the standard methods for toxicological studies related to drug safety for applications for approval and to serve for the appropriate evaluation of drug safety.

However, it is not always reasonable to apply a unified method for all drugs, and it often becomes necessary to perform additional new tests during the course of the study. Therefore, the experimental methods noted here are not intended to be strictly followed as long as the data obtained are useful for safety evaluation for clinical applications.

1. Acute, Subacute and Chronic Toxicity Studies

In principle, toxicity studies with both rodents and non-rodents should be conducted on every new drug. According to the period of clinical application, the administration period of test drugs in each toxicity study is as follows in principle.

	Administration Frequency or Period		
Period of Clinical Application	Acute Toxicity	Subacute Toxicity	Chronic Toxicity
Drugs to be administered Once	Once	28 days	Not Required
Drugs to be administered for One Week or Less	Once	90 days	Not Required
Drugs to be administered Exceeding One Week and up to Four Weeks	Once	28 days	6 months
Drugs to be administered for Over Four Weeks	Once	90 days	1 year

* Such as acute, subacute and chronic toxicity studies in each species, reproduction I, II and III studies in each species, and mutagenicity I, II and III studies and carcinogenicity studies in each species.

1. Studies with Rodents

a) Experimental Animals
   - Species and strains of experimental animals should be selected in consideration of life span spontaneous disease incidence, sensitivity to know toxic substances and other factors.
   - When acute, subacute, and chronic toxicity studies are performed on a substance, it is desirable that animals of the same species and strain be used.
b) Experimental Methods
   - Acute Toxicity Study
   a) Animals: At least 2 species of healthily grown adult animals of both sexes should be used (Note 1).
   b) Number of animals: Groups should consist of at least 5 animals of each sex.
   c) Administration route: In principle, oral and parenteral administration routes, including the expected clinical route, should be employed (Notes 2 and 3). If the expected clinical route is special and not applicable to the animals, other appropriate routes should be employed.
   d) Dose levels: Sufficient numbers of dose groups should be employed for determination of LD50 values for each sex in principle (Notes 4 and 5).
   e) Administration: Administration should be single in principle.
   f) Observation period: The observation period should be 2 weeks in principle.
   g) Experimental Procedure:
      - General signs of all the animals in each group should be observed daily, and body weights be measured at least 3 times during the observation period.
      - At the termination of the observation period (or at the time of death), all animals in each group should be autopsied and gross observations should be made on organs and tissues (Note 6). Organ weight measurement and histopathological examinations should be performed on the organs with gross alterations, if necessary.

2. Studies with Non-rodents

a) Experimental Animals
   When acute, subacute, and chronic toxicity studies are performed in series on a substance, it is desirable that animals of the same species be used throughout the studies.
b) Experimental Method
   - Acute Toxicity Study
   a) Animals: At least 1 species of animals should be used (Note 1).
   b) Number of animals: Groups should consist of at least 2 animals.
   c) Administration route: The administration should be in accordance with the expected clinical route in principle (Note 2).
   d) Dose levels: At least 2 dose groups sufficient for determination of the approximate lethal dose should be employed (Note 5).
   e) Administration: Administration should be single, in principle.

f) Observation period: The observation period should be 2 weeks, in principle.
g) Experimental Procedure:
   1. All animals in each group should be observed for general appearance daily and body weights measured at least 3 times during the observation period. Clinical laboratory tests should be performed if necessary.
   2. At the termination of the observation period (or at the time of death), all animals in each group should be autopsied and gross observations should be made on organs and tissues (Note 6). Further, if necessary, organ weight measurement and histopathological examinations should be performed on main organs and tissues.

Notes

Note 1 Generally, mice and rats are used as rodents, and dogs and monkeys as non-rodents.

Note 2 Oral administration should be made by gavage in principle. In that case, the animals should be fasted usually for a certain time before administration of the substance.

Note 3 In the case of parenteral administration, it is desirable to employ at least 2 routes of administration.

Note 4 Generally, at least 5 groups are employed, and the LD50 value is calculated by probit method, etc.

Note 5 If the toxicity of the substance is too low to determine the lethal dose, a technically applicable maximum dose should be employed as the highest dose.

Note 6 Gross observations should be made on all the organs and tissues.

Acute toxicity testing is a simple but indispensable procedure for the assessment and evaluation of the toxic characteristics of a drug. It is usually conducted as the first step in the various toxicological and pharmacological experiments required in full development of a medicine.

The acute toxicity test is designed to clarify the adverse effects of a drug on animals occuring after administration of a single dose. In this type of test it is necessary carefully to observe and record, the type, extent and duration of the toxic signs, their progression and the occurence of death for two or more weeks after the dose. The signs of toxicity to be assessed include changes in posture, locomotor activity, respiratory and circulatory activities and body temperature, as well as effects due to an action on the autonomic and central nervous system, such as tremors, convulsions, paralysis, salivation or lethargy. Change in body weight, diet and water consumption may provide further information on the toxic effects of the drug.

Naked-eye and microscopic examination of organ and tissues in animals who die or are sacrificed may give useful information on the mode of toxicity. Biochemical examinations may also give information about the mechanism of action. From the mortality at each dosage level, the LD50 value of the drug should be estimated.

The term, "acute toxicity test" tends to be used as a synonym for "acute lethality test" or "LD50 test", but it must be realized that we expect to get extensive information on the toxicological characteristics of the drug as well as the LD50 value. The acute toxicity test is suitable for obtaining toxicological information about acute overdosage, since other toxicological tests mentioned in the Toxicity Test Guideline are repeat dosing studies.

The data obtained from acute toxicity test may be utilized as follows:

1. The data may be used as dose-finding information for subacute and chronic toxicity studies, and in toxicokinetic and pharmacological studies. The clinical pharmacologist may also refer to the data in planning Phase I clinical trials.
2. In the regulatory agency, the data are used for assessment and evaluation of the acute toxic potential of the drug and for considering intoxication due to overdosage or an accident.

In our Toxicity Test Guideline, the acute toxicity test is required as a standard procedure, in which 5 male and 5 female rodents and 2 non-rodents are used at each dosage level.

The LD50 for rodents will be calculated exactly utilizing a standard statistical method, but for nonrodents, which are used in small numbers, only an approximate value is determined. In acute toxicity tests in non-rodents, emphasis and priority should be placed on the observation of toxic signs and the course of the intoxication induced by the drug.

We are deeply interested in the development of alternative methods using fewer animals for the estimation of the LD50 and in their scientific validation, since no alternative method has yet been authorized by the government of any country. Much attention is being paid to the various procedures that have recently been proposed, because they either employ fewer animals to obtain acute toxicity data or because they are designed to minimise the number of animals required to measure the LD50.

During preparation of the Japanese Acute Toxicity Test Guideline, drafts for comment were sent to the authorities in the European Community and the USA. The replies were discussed in working groups and some of the comments were adopted to attain methodological harmonisation with the requirements in those countries.

At present the Japanese Toxicity Test Guideline may be regarded as comparable to the OECD test Guideline and similar guidelines in the toxicity requirements of other countries.

All animal experiments in Japan have to be performed in accordance with the requirements for the protection and control of animals.

Discussion following Dr. Crawford, Dr. Tezuka and Dr. Takanaka

PROF. ZBINDEN:

Why does the national guideline require acute studies in two species by two routes of a medicine intended for oral administration to man.

DR. TAKANAKA:

The acute toxicity test is usually done in the first steps of development of a drug and was used to check toxicity. Industry would often wish to use the drug for oral administration first, but if approval was obtained, application would be made for other routes, making it important to obtain more information about the toxic characteristics of each drug. There may be some difference between routes, the signs of toxicity may differ between routes, and LD50 values are sometimes different in males and females. The results may give information about the pharmacokinetics of the drugs or the effect of drug metabolising enzymes.

PROF. DAYAN:

It is possible to do studies in non-rodents in which the pharmacodynamic responses to high doses are closely monitored, but without extending the treatment as far as a lethal dose. How acceptable would this type of pharmacological experimentation be to the Japanese authorities?

DR. TAKANAKA:

Before clinical trials, sufficient information is required to predict safety in use. Observations should be made up to the approximate lethal dose in non-rodent animals. Precise LD50's were not required, only a minimum lethal dose or a maximum tolerated dose.

PROF. ZBINDEN:

Would a limit test be acceptable, and if so, what would be the limit?

DR. TAKANAKA:

No general answer could be given and there would be case by case consideration of each substance. The Japanese guideline does not mention a fixed upper limit to the dosage to be examined for a new medicinal preparation. We are interested in Japan in the impetus in other countries that a limit test be adopted and we may consider it in Japan.

Dr. Takanaka was asked about how many animals would be required in each group in an LD50 test.

He replied that the guideline stated "sufficient numbers for the statistical evaluation". At the start of an experiment no one can know how many animals may be needed to achieve a statistically significant difference. It is for that reason that "sufficient numbers" is mentioned. Researchers are asked to establish the appropriate group size from knowledge gained during the experiments.

There was interest in knowing the attitude of the Japanese and US authorities to drugs to be given to young children. Was it necessary for regulatory purposes to include acute toxicity data in newborn animals?

It was agreed by Dr. Takanaka that the Japanese guidelines did include a requirement for acute toxicity testing in weanling animals. This was necessary because different responses sometimes occurred in young and adult animals, due to differences in drug metabolising capacity etc. Weanlings were preferred to neonatal animals.

Dr. Takanaka stated that it was difficult to extrapolate from neonatal animals to children, but it was still considered important to do such tests, because they added to the overall knowledge of the actions of the drug, and might give some indication to the mechanism of its toxic effects.

Dr. Takanaka was asked about public opinion and animal experimentation in Japan. He replied that in Japan the animal welfare groups were not powerful. The Japanese have a long history of caring for animals and strong feelings for their protection, although the public in general knows little about experimentation.

A questioner asked about the requirement in the Japanese guideline for a study in large animals. Dr. Takanaka explained that the need for and the nature of the study could only be decided by consideration of the properties of individual compounds as they were reviewed.

A final statement from the floor referred to the importance of adapting statistical techniques to the nature of the biological experiment being analysed. It was conceivable that more useful data for extrapolation might be obtained from small animals if doses were expressed allometrically, i.e. in relation to body surface area rather than just to weight.

Alternatives to Animals in Toxicological Assessment and Notifications

V. H. Morgenroth

Introduction

The OECD is an international organisation established in 1960. Its origins lie in the Organisation for European Economic Cooperation, which was established in 1948 to administer funds from the Marshall Plan. Its Member countries includes 24 industrialised countries from Western Europe, the Far East, Australia and North America. In chemicals production and trade, these countries account for in excess of 70% of commerce.

In the late '60s, the Member countries concluded that greater consideration should be given to the quality of economic cooperation and development. One fundamental aspect of this was concern for the state of the environment which provides the ecological basis for all economic activities.

In the early 1970s, the OECD Member countries noted that almost any chemical has a potential to be hazardous and therefore merits scrutiny for environmental and health effects before being used. Thus, one of the primary goals that had been clearly identified in the Member countries and therefore addressed under the OECD Chemicals Programme, is improved and cost-effective protection of man and the environment from the potential harmful effects of chemicals. In the same countries, the goal of promoting the welfare of animals used for experimental purposes has also been assigned a high priority.

Recently, the Second High Level Meeting of the Chemicals Group attended by Ministers and high level administrators responsible for chemicals control in the 24 Member countries issued a statement concerning the relationships between the work of the OECD Chemicals Programme and Animal Welfare.

- "The welfare of laboratory animals is important. It will continue to be an important factor influencing the work in the OECD Chemicals Programme, and the progress in OECD on the harmonization of chemicals control, in particular the agreement on Mutual Acceptance of Data, by looking at the number of animals, and reducing the number used in testing. Such testing cannot be eliminated at present, but every effort should be made to discover, develop and validate alternative testing systems."
- "The High Level Meeting invites the Chemicals Group, the Management Committee, the Updating Panel, lead countries and the Secretariat, to ensure that the spirit of this declaration is an integral part of their work."

OECD Chemicals Programme and Animal Welfare

Thus, the consideration of animal welfare is also an explicit goal of the work of the OECD Chemicals Programme. What is the relationship between the goals of protecting man and the environment and the welfare of laboratory animals? Clearly, to protect man's environment includes the protection of birds, mammals, fish, etc. But to attain such a goal, it is necessary to have sufficient information available to assess the potential hazards of a chemical. In other words, a certain number of laboratory animals have to be sacrificed in order to protect man and animals. We can query whether more information on the effects of certain chlorinated pesticides would have kept the peregrine falcon off the endangered species list, or whether we can safely treat a number of animal maladies such as heart worms with new drugs without assessing the potential hazards of such drugs? Animal testing has been and will continue to be for some future time, one of the methods employed to gain this essential information. Is this incompatible with the promotion of animal welfare? The answer to the question of the relationship between the two goals seems to be one of balance. Testing yes, but only that which is necessary to gain the essential information necessary to protect man and the environment.

Do internationally agreed means exist by which the amount of testing can be effectively reduced, thus affecting the numbers of animals used, and further what can be done to improve the welfare of test animals where this sacrifice is presently unavoidable? Let's examine one product of the OECD Chemicals Programme.

Decision on Mutual Acceptance of Data

In 1981, the OECD Council adopted a Decision on the Mutual Acceptance of Data which is stated as follows:

"Test data on a chemical generated in one Member country in accordance with the OECD Test Guidelines and the OECD Principles of Good Laboratory Practice, shall be accepted in other Member countries for purposes of assessment and other uses relating to the protection of man and the environment."

This decision means that if test data on chemical "X" are generated in Country "A" according to a method described in one of the OECD Test Guidelines and in accord with the OECD Principles of Good Laboratory Practice, and if Country "B" also needs the same test data, chemical "X" does not have to be re-tested. Therefore, the implementation of this Decision by Member countries will significantly reduce the duplicative testing of chemicals. It will result in more effective utilisation of scarce test facilities and specialist manpower, and it certainly will reduce significantly the total number of animals used in testing. The Guidelines (at present covering more than fifty test parameters) and the Principles of Good Laboratory Practice annexed to the Decision provide the first internationally agreed upon procedures for testing of chemicals. This Decision is legally binding only for the OECD Member countries but, in fact, these Guidelines are being used on a much broader international scale.

An examination of the Test Guidelines themselves provides a further insight into a means of reducing the number of animals tested. In the preamble section to the Health Effects Guidelines, it is stated:

"for the objective of an efficient approach to testing chemicals there is no point in having more groups or more animals per group than are strictly necessary to attain the end-point of the reliable detection of toxic effects."

This consideration is reflected in a number of the Health Effects Guidelines. For example, the number of animals recommended per group in the Acute, Repeated-dose, Subchronic, Irritancy Guidelines are all lower than for methods previously applied. In fact, several guidelines reduce by half the numbers of animals per group, but are still statistically adequate to measure the desired toxicological end-points. In nine of the short and intermediate duration Health Effects Guidelines a "limit test" is described. This "limit test" recommends that if at test at *one* high dose level, using the procedures described for the study, produces no test chemical related effects, then a full study using three dose levels may be considered unnecessary. This "limit test" serves to delineate the presence or absence of toxic hazards from the test compound. This new concept introduced in the OECD Test Guidelines is particularly important in reducing the number of animals needed to assess those substances likely to be toxic only under conditions of high exposure levels.

The OECD Test Guidelines for the determination of the possible irritant or corrosive effects of a chemical recommend that chemicals known to be strongly acidic, alkaline or toxic should not be tested. Rather than the results of animal testing, these properties would be used to indicate the possible hazard from dermal or ocular exposure to the chemical. Further, substances shown to irritate skin are not recommended to be tested in the eye. Thus, the total number of chemicals tested is reduced. These last recommendations in the Guidelines illustrate another important consideration in the testing of chemicals that is, that the welfare of the animals that have to be used in testing should be protected to the greatest extent possible. Or in the words of the Test Guidelines:

"Stringent control of environmental conditions and proper animal care techniques are mandatory."

Furthermore, one of the Test Guidelines describes procedures for the use of local anesthetics if the test chemical is suspected of having the potential to cause pain to the test animal. The OECD Principles of Good Laboratory Practice, the other annex to the Decision on Mutual Acceptance of Data, also makes a number of recommendations concerning the welfare test animals. For example, it is stated that proper conditions should be established and maintained for the housing, handling and care of animals. In addition, it is stated that:

"conditions should comply with appropriate national regulatory requirements for the import, collection, care and use of animals ..."

In conclusion, the OECD Decision on the Mutual Acceptance of Data taken by the OECD Member countries demonstrates a number of the means by which the goal of protecting man and the environment from the harmful effect of chemicals can be balanced with the goal of promoting animal welfare.

OECD Chemicals Programme on Alternative Methodology

Before closing, I would like to consider a new initiative in the area of alternative methodology being undertaken by the OECD Member countries under the OECD Chemicals Programme. It has been pointed out that there are good correlations between the results of short term *in-vitro* mutagenicity tests and the carcinogenic potential of chemicals. Further, a number of these short term *in-vitro* screening tests are being used in OECD Member countries to screen for and identify potential mammalian carcinogens. Test Guidelines for some of these tests are currently under review by various policy bodies within the OECD. In fact, four Test Guidelines are in the final stage of this review process and will hopefully be adopted as OECD Test Guidelines in the near future. These four guidelines will then represent the first internationally agreed mutually acceptable approach to alternative *in-vitro* methods for screening chemicals for potential carcinogenic effects.

Other activities of the OECD Chemicals Programme impacting on the protection of animal welfare include: work in the area of information exchange, harmonization of criteria for selecting chemicals for further study, harmonization of principles of hazard assessment as well as the Updating of OECD Test Guidelines which is designed to identify and develop guidelines for alternative and new testing methodology.

Certainly the developments occurring in the fields of "alternative methodology" are exciting and offer the prospect of not only saving animals but of increasing our ability and resource capability for assessing the potential hazards of chemicals. There is a growing body of knowledge on the usefulness of alternative methodologies (including test methods, structure-activity relationships and the use of computer estimations and simulation) which is being closely followed by the OECD Chemicals Programme. However, it is important to remember that most of these developments are still at an early stage and at present the need remains to evaluate chemicals on the basis of laboratory study and testing. Therefore, efforts which reduce the total number of tests performed through international cooperation, information sharing, harmonization of chemicals management, and stimulation of research and application of alternative methods offer an important means to promote animal welfare in the context of maintaining adequate protection of man and the environment.

In summary, at present the testing of chemicals is necessary if we are to protect the public health and our environment, but this testing should be done in ways that minimise numbers of animals used and which take full account of their welfare. The drive to develop alternatives must include the analysis of the validity, extrapolability and consequences of the use of such methods. The demand for greater assurance of the safety of the chemicals we use and animal welfare can and must be balanced. Approaches must be sought that ensure that progress toward these goals can be achieved. One such approach is being undertaken by the Member countries of OECD through their Chemicals Programme. The results and work of this Programme have significantly affected in a positive way the welfare of laboratory animals and the numbers of animals used in testing and it will continue to do so in the future.

Summary

The major goals motivating the work under the OECD Chemicals Programme are: improving the protection of man and the environment from potential harmful effects of chemicals, avoiding potential non-tariff barriers to trade in chemicals, and facilitating the economically efficient and scientifically sound management of chemicals among member countries, particularly in the areas of testing methodology, good laboratory practice, and information exchange. The results obtained from the work have clear benefits to both government and industry, not the least in terms of conserving scarce resources – including laboratory animals. Both the number of animals needed in testing and the welfare of laboratory animals have been and will be significantly affected in a positive way. The results and work of the OECD Chemicals Programme are presented emphasising the impact on animal welfare and the development of alternative methodologies.

Discussion following Dr. Morgenroth

The political and administrative measures required to amend national or international regulations take many months to be completed. As a result, changes in the science of toxicology are often a very long time ahead of alterations in its regulatory practices.

Toxicologists working in the laboratory can gain much valuable information about the properties and effects of substances, especially novel compounds, by doing limited exploratory single dose tests, in which many variables are examined. This type of experiment is much closer to pharmacological than to classical single dose toxicity testing, but its flexibility and scope are now making it more generally attractive. Within the development of a pharmaceutical, however, it still comprises only a very small proportion of the data available, and even in the case of an industrial chemical, say, additional biological information is likely to be made available when safety is being assessed.

In any acute toxicity experiment, it is advisable to make a wide range of clinical observations including, when appropriate, measurement of heart and respiratory rate, and changes in other physiological systems, and a detailed autopsy. Histopathological studies are likely to be worthwhile only if sufficient time has elapsed for morphological changes to develop.

The spacing, timing and routes of doses were discussed, but without an unanimous conclusion being reached. It was agreed that several, spaced doses should be employed, but it was not certain whether they could be administered to separate animals concurrently or consecutively. The oral and a parenteral route should be employed for most pharmaceuticals.

Biologicals, such as vaccines and sera, should not be regarded in the same way as chemicals. Simple, acute dose studies have been valuable in helping to produce safe preparations, but their importance is being reduced.

III. Summary Reports of Group Discussions

Introductory Comments on Ethical Aspects of Acute Toxicity Testing

A. D. Dayan

The ethics of acute studies of this type include general considerations at the philosophical level of the morality of experiments that involve animals, and specific and more utilitarian examination of the need to employ them in acute toxicity studies.

The general philosophical problem has been debated for several thousand years. Inheritors of the Judaeo-Christian tradition have analysed the statement in the Bible attributing to man dominion over all living creatures and have generally come to accept the view that dominion is limited by moral constraints, especially the importance of avoiding cruelty and suffering. Greek and Renaissance philosophers subsequently reassessed the general relationship of man to animals, their views tending to reflect an increasing personalisation and humanitarianism in the relationship of man to man and man to state. This tendency has continued to the present as various nineteenth and twentieth century scholars have futher developed concepts of individual responsibility and social organisation, culminating in such political ideas as fascism and racism. The attempt by a few to develop as a parallel concept speciesism, ie. that animals have rights quite identical to those of man, has met with general diasagreement, because it requires the attribution to animals of sentience and spiritual powers for which there is no acceptable evidence.

Nonetheless, developments in moral and ethical thinking have repeatedly stressed the need for kindness and sympathy towards all species, lest the sensitivity of man himself be impaired by the cruelty and suffering of others.

At the pragmatic level, there is ample evidence to show the inestimable value of toxicity testing in the safer development and use of medicines, pesticides and many other products of modern industries. The question that now arises, given that there is ethical justification in principle for animal studies, is the circumstances and the extent to which acute toxicity testing is morally acceptable.

From the utilitarian view point, the moral scientist considering an acute toxicity experiment should first ask in what way are the data important in advancing knowledge, whether of normal body processes or of the properties of a specific compound, or of a particular medicine or other product.

Once he has decided that there is justifiable purpose in the proposed study, which includes being certain that the information is necessary and that it cannot be obtained in any other way, then there is a further series of questions to be answered satisfactorily before the experiment can be done. They are: what types of data are required, are the skills and equipment needed to make those observations available and applicable to the minimum number of animals, and do knowledge and experience show that excessive pain or suffering will not be caused to the animals involved?

In practice, these linked questions include several considerable areas of experimental design and analysis to obtain the maximum usable information from the smallest number of animals and to attain proper husbandry and experimental technique. They also cover the ethical responsibilities of the individual scientist and his professional and technical colleagues in ensuring that the highest professional standards are maintained at the same time as care and compassion are exercised.

The acute toxicity test is ethically acceptable as a limited experiment involving a small number of animals, following a carefully thought out design, and done to gain important knowledge to protect man and other animals.

The formal LD50 test, however, as generally understood, must usually be regarded with suspicion as often providing unnecessary and unreliable results from an excessive number of animals. If assessment of the scientific requirements does not show real need for the special type of quantitative data it provides, then the LD50 test must be regarded as unethical.

Consideration of the academic need for and practical uses made of the results of acute toxicity testing show that it is only in a few special instances that it is essential or at least helpful to have precise LD50 data rather than an account of the spectrum of acute toxicity.

Scientific Constraints on the Use of Acute Toxicity Testing

A. D. Dayan (Chairman)

B. B. Newbould (Rapporteur)

I experienced excitement and elation at the common sense shown by contributors, but also depression over the length of time needed to change things. Our session had a rigorous discussion on *the more scientific aspects of constraints on the use of acute toxicity testing*.

It was generally accepted that there might reasonably be a difference in protocols for acute toxicity tests between pharmaceuticals, including pesticides and agrochemicals (small part of larger package of data), and general chemicals, where they formed a larger part of a smaller package of information. However, we were reminded that having embarked on an acute test, no matter what the design, if the job was worth doing it was worth doing properly.

We touched on biologicals, e.g. vaccine and sera, and noted with satisfaction that bioassays of the type conceived by Trevan had largely fallen into disuse, as they had been replaced by immune assays, etc. The scientists urged those concerned with regulations to continue to look critically at the remaining acute toxicity tests which appeared to form part of pharmaceutical requirements.

In considering the *design* of acute toxicity experiments, we did not attempt to define the ideal protocol, but it became quite clear that toxicologists had a key role in designing experiments which were likely to yield the maximum amount of information with the minimum of use of animals. That is, toxicologists must move towards being experimental biologists rather than just "tickers-off" of boxes in a check list. There were no universal rules at this stage on whether to start high and then to reduce the doses in general acute experiments, or vice versa, or what dose spacing should be used, but there was general agreement that careful thought was required. Some expressed reservations about the value of studying multiple routes of exposure for a new pharmaceutical intended only to be given by mouth. There was general agreement that i. p. dosing was irrelevant in safety assessment of pharmaceuticals.

Many contributions to the discussion made it clear that much could be learned by *careful observation* of effects on the behaviour of animals in experiments, number of stools passed, colour of skin, rate of breathing, etc. *Histology* too has an important part to play under the right circumstances, particularly when careful observation at necropsy has indicated that a particular organ looks abnormal. Measures of biochemical parameters are not generally regarded as particularly useful at present, but further research may reveal their value.

It was interesting to reflect on Dr. Volan's contribution yesterday, in which he regarded the results of acute toxicity tests in animals as of limited value to a practising physician in charge of a Poisons Centre. However, it is important to recognize that these remarks related to medicaments on trial or sale rather than compounds at an early stage of development. One discussant placed the value of acute tests in the latter circumstance as below those of dose ranging studies conducted over several days.

Practical Constraints on the Use of Acute Toxicity Testing

F. CLEMENTI (Chairman)

J. M. FRAZIER (Rapporteur)

The objective of this discussion group was to comment on the practical problems associated both with current acute toxicity testing procedures and proposed alternatives methods. Initial discussions focussed on the problem of large variability in data both between and within laboratories conducting acute toxicity testing. The order of magnitude difference in reported LD50's between laboratories was cited as a case in point. The following are some generalized summaries of the group's comments on current testing procedures:

a) There was a general feeling that large variation in LD50s were not a practical problem, since regulatory authorities seldom questioned and/or commented on LD50s unless they indicated extremely toxic substances, which would not be certified under any conditions.
b) There was concern that experimental variability could be manipulated by selection of species, vehicle, etc. to produce the most favorable results. However, it was pointed out by the regulatory side that such manipulations were well known and could not ultimately influence the review of a drug.
c) Furthermore, from a regulatory point of view, where large variability between sets of acute toxicity data exists, significant efforts are made to determine the nature of the variability, i.e. is it due to species differences, routes of administration, diets, laboratory procedures, etc.?

Next, there was some discussion of practical problems associated with non-*in vitro* alternatives, for example tests which used fewer animals but involved extensive observations. The following comments were presented:

a) One problem with alternatives which involve extensive observations is an apparent need for additional personnel. These individuals will most likely be technicians and will require additional training. Observational data by technicians will have to be accepted under Good Laboratory Practices (GLP) regulations, and will probably require a precise vocabulary of terms to describe observations. Such procedures will probably prove expensive.
b) It was observed that, unlike drugs which undergo extensive clinical trials before introduction into the consumer market, other industrial chemicals cannot be so tested. Such data are available only after the products are on the market and usually are evaluated by poison control units as accidental exposures and suicide attempts.

With respect to *in vitro* approaches to acute toxicity testing, the following comments were presented:

a) It was generally agreed that from a practical point of view it will be some time before *in vitro* methods can completely replace whole animal acute toxicity testing in the drug industry. Whole animal acute toxicity tests are of significant value to the industry because of the scientific information generated concerning presentation of symptoms and the time course of responses, as well as the development of treatments for acute toxicity. However, it was felt that significantly fewer animals were required for these research purposes than are necessary for a GLP-LD50 test.
b) There was significant concern that a battery of *in vitro* tests designed to replace whole animal toxicity testing would be an economic burden. The key problems being:
the need for highly trained technical personnel to conduct such tests,
the requirements for sophisticated analytical instrumentation, and
adequate facilities for cell culture work.
c) The question of inter-laboratory variability was raised with respect to *in vitro* testing systems. Historically, the problem with obtaining reproducible results with the Ames' mutagenicity test is of concern. The experience of FRAME (Fund for the Replacement of Animals in Medical Experimentation) was enlightening, since it demonstrated that careful attention to details and standardized protocols can significantly reduce inter-laboratory variability for *in vitro* tests.
d) It was generally felt that in the near future the role of *in vitro* methods would be complementary to whole animal tests and that the real value of *in vitro* systems is to study mechanisms of action of toxic substances.

As a last point of discussion, the group was asked to consider under what condition would an LD50 measurement be of value. Several suggestions were considered:

a) For some of the most toxic anti-neoplastic drugs which are taken at high dosages an LD50 bioassay may be required for quality control.
b) In development of rodenticides, LD50s are needed to evaluate efficacy.
c) A precise LD50 is probably not required for antidote research.
d) For studies of structure-activity relationships for series of related compounds accurate LD50s may be needed.
e) Finally, the LD50 may be required for quality control of some antibiotics.

Regulatory Constraints on the Use of Acute Toxicity Testing

G. FÜLGRAFF (Chairman)

A. STEIGER (Rapporteur)

The group reviewed regulatory constraints and influences on the use of acute toxicity data. First it considered existing requirements at the national and international levels. Several difficulties and conflicts were identified. The balance between animal welfare and the health of man; differences between aspects of large multi-national industries and smaller industries; conflicts between guidelines for drugs and those for chemicals; and last, differing views in various nations.

Second, a large degree of harmony has now been achieved with regard to acute toxicity testing within Europe – the EEC and North America – the FDA and HPB.

Third, the classical (formal) LD50 test is still required in Japan and a qualitatively similar and more narrowly defined test is still set out in the OECD guidelines. That means a test with five animals of each sex in six dose groups.

Fourth, it is recognised that OECD has an influential role in fostering international harmonization, but it is important for individual countries to decide definitely whether or not their guidelines for testing chemicals are to be applied to pharmaceuticals, too. They must also ensure that their procedures for updating guidelines are streamlined to the point where they can have a positive influence on national and regional policies. It appears that OECD proposals will probably be discussed in the near future by the Updating Panel of the Management Committee. Various procedures such as the up-down procedure, the fixed dose procedure and other methods of replacing the classical LD50 test will be considered.

Fifth, it is important that the industry itself should have a voice in determining policy at national and international levels, although there may be constraints in achieving this, since companies are in competition with each other.

Sixth, in the interests of a unified policy by industry, it is of great importance that there be an independent, international forum for representatives of industry, regulatory bodies and academia to discuss issues and to enable responses to be taken rapidly. If this is not done, industry is open to the criticism that it is doing too little too late.

Last, toxicology in any case is in constant evolution and methods such as those discussed here must always be adequately justified on scientific grounds at national, regional and international levels.

IFPMA – A View on Acute Toxicity Testing in Relation to Pharmaceuticals

R. Arnold

I am pleased to have the opportunity to present to you today an industry view on acute toxicity testing.

I must preface my remarks by saying that I know I am talking with a little acquired knowledge, to a group of experts in the field of animal toxicology, in which I have no expertise whatsoever, but because what I say will be part of the record of the meeting, I feel obliged to mention a number of elementary points, which will be well known to you, but less so perhaps to a wider and less specialized readership.

The widespread interest in the issue of animal experimentation makes it very probable that the proceedings of this conference will be widely read and I hope therefore that today's audience will understand the reasons for some of my remarks today.

You have heard both yesterday and this morning a comprehensive review of the various aspects of acute toxicity testing. Such studies play a small but essential role in the preclinical assessment of a chemical substance in laboratory animals. The pharmaceutical industry has long taken the view that formal LD50 determinations, which require large numbers of animals, are rarely necessary. I am pleased that the presentations from various regulatory bodies have shown that this view is also taken by the authorities responsible for marketing authorizations of new drug substances.

Although both Dr. Oliver and Dr. Morgenroth have presented views in relation to industrial chemicals, I should like to confine my comments to the toxicological assessment of a pharmaceutical as a part of its safety evaluation. We cannot ignore the fact that pharmaceuticals also require safety evaluation as industrial chemicals and the meeting has been helpful in clarifying the way in which acute toxicity data can be generally used in classification of industrial chemicals.

Investigations of all aspects of the potential toxicity of any new drug substance are conducted in order to evaluate possible adverse effects in use in man. Information about the effects of a single dose of a substance has become traditionally identified with a formal LD50 determination about which Professor Zbinden has already spoken.

This expression has subsequently become very widely used to define acute toxicity. This "formal" LD50 is often confused with other acute toxicity determinations and it has been pointed out we must ensure that these concepts remain separate. However, the level of statistical precision implied by the formal method is rarely justified as the data obtained from different experiments in different laboratories using different strains of animal have been shown to give widely varying results. A study conducted by Hunter in 1979 for the Commission of the European Communities in a number of European countries has demonstrated this very effectively.

I believe that our discussions over the last two days have shown the reasons behind these variations and they have certainly been very comprehensively reviewed by our first speaker, Professor Zbinden (see p. 5 ff.). It has been shown that approximate LD50 values obtained from dose ranging studies are just as likely to be valid in a statistical sense as formal values. Dr. Schütz and others, for example Lork, have shown that there is excellent agreement between conventional LD50 determinations and LD50s calculated by re-analysis of the same data using a smaller number of animals. Thus, acute toxicity can be assessed without using a large number of animals.

I think it is helpful to remind you again of the range of acute toxicity studies which can be conducted and to re-emphasize the distinction between the limitations of the formal LD50 determination and the flexibility of other studies conducted.

First, but now increasingly rarely a "formal" LD50 determination can be made.

Second, a limit test can be used, that is a study in which small numbers of animals are used per group. Only a small number of doses are given, which do not exceed a pre-set "limit" dose, the maximum employed even if it does not induce any acute effects.

Third, a range of other procedures based on "up-down" and other ranging methods, in which very small numbers of animals are dosed. At the first indication of an effect, a further larger group is tested at a lower dose level. A number of new approaches of this type have been used and some have been described earlier in this meeting.

Fourth, *in vitro* methods are being developed to replace the acute toxicity study. As yet no satisfactory way has been found to mimic the complex inter-related responses obtained in acute studies in whole animals, however, further research in this area may prove such methods to be a useful adjunct in the future.

The use of acute toxicity observations in the development of pharmaceuticals is essential and varied. It ranges from the very early assessment of a new substance before administration to man through to potency testing of certain vaccines. An essential part of these studies is to investigate the pharmacodynamic changes following the single dose and data from these studies may be used to set dose levels in repeated dose animal studies and perhaps in early human studies. Small numbers of rodents and often non-rodents are used to explore a range of effects which normally does not include lethality.

These data would certainly be used in association with other information, e.g. from pharmacokinetic studies. All of this evidence is generated at a very early stage in the development of a pharmaceutical and it is unlikely to be necessary to repeat it at any later point.

Dr. Volans has already reviewed the need for some indication of doses at which poisoning may occur. This is of particular concern in relation to children and such data are necessary for the investigation of antidotes.

It is clear that the uses of acute toxicity data are wide. It is one of the most readily accessible and widely adopted pieces of information known about a substance, particularly in relation to an industrial chemical. Professor Dayan has indicated the need for careful consideration of the ethical aspects of any laboratory animal study. Acute toxicity testing in the form of the LD50 determination has always been a contentious subject. For many years safety evaluation scientists within the pharmaceutical industry have been anxious to minimize the use of these studies because of the ethical concerns they raise.

An acute toxicity study is at risk of causing suffering in laboratory animals, and thus such a study must be embarked upon in a very responsible manner so as to reduce the number of animals used and to ensure that they yield the maximum amount of useful information. I believe that your discussions over the last two days do indicate the critical importance of acute toxicity data in the overall safety evaluation of a new drug substance. The discussions have also underlined the fact that scientists both in industry and in regulatory authorities are well aware of their responsibilities and keen to generate and use these data in the best possible way. The use of the formal LD50 will be minimized in the future and acute toxicity studies will be employed within a proper context to provide necessary information. To this end, the pharmaceutical industry has agreed a series of recommendations which we feel will help to guide scientists conducting such studies. They are: –

1. The determination of "formal" LD50 values for pharmaceuticals should be limited to the very few cases when other methods for assessment of acute toxicity will not suffice.
2. The maximum amount of relevant information about the acute toxicity of a substance should be obtained, using the minimum number of animals in the most humane way possible.
3. Non-rodent animals, such as dogs, should be used only for assessment of acute toxicity as a part of dose ranging studies, where lethality is not the end point.
4. Regulatory authorities, internationally, should be flexible in their approach to the requirement for acute toxicity data on drugs and help to avoid unnecessary repetition of studies to fulfil national regulatory obligations.

It is often difficult to reach an agreed position between colleagues in one organization. It is more difficult to do so between workers in different organizations in the same country. It has given me particular satisfaction therefore that there has been such unanimity of view between industry scientists at an international level, so that the IFPMA Position Paper has been based on genuine agreement rather than compromise.

The issue of animal experimentation has become an important ethical issue in many countries, among which, of course, Switzerland and the U.K. come readily to mind. The public at large may not always realize that the industry more than any group wishes to minimise the use of animals in research and testing. But, of course, to achieve this, we must at the same time preserve the standards of safety and efficacy which industry and society as a whole consider necessary. These standards are given tangible form in the requirements of governmental drug regulatory authorities. Any moves to reduce the number of animals must depend on acceptance of the latter. I am very pleased that the discussions over the past two days, which have brought together experts from industry and from the regulatory agencies, have been a step in the right direction.

Closing Remarks

G. FÜLGRAFF (Chairman)

May I begin my summary by quoting one phrase from Professor Zbinden's presentation yesterday. He said, referring to the assessment of acute toxicity, that, "We can do better than we have done in the past". I think this is the main appeal of this conference, to do better with respect to acute toxicity testing. That means to elaborate an acute toxicity profile of new substances with a flexible approach adequate to the substance and to the purpose of the investigation, instead of just applying a general experimental scheme. This appeal is directed to all of us, in industry, as well as in drug control agencies.

To introduce such a change, conferences like this are certainly more helpful than the frequent complaints about bureaucracies in one organization or other. As a matter of fact these complaints are often justified. We register from time to time bureaucratic attitudes in authorities as well as in industrial companies. These two bureaucracies even sustain each other; they need each other, one being the condition for the importance of the other. Any intended change is a process of mutual adaptation or education under the watchful eyes of a suspicious public.

The protection of human and animal health and environment lies in the responsibility of many parts of society, but in particular legislators and government are responsible for protecting public health. Their decisions are based on information provided by scientific investigations, but the decisions are not scientific in themselves. Hence the information needed by those who make decisions is particularly critical; it must allow us to end with a valid risk/benefit-evaluation which is always the case for regulatory decisions.

A critical scientist working for government continously questions the validity of the regulation he enforces; together with politicians, he will try to improve regulations and to overcome the comfortable tendency to continue with once-established rules and procedures. As I said before, this tendency is widespread and to be found not only in state authorities.

There are at least three reasons which make it necessary continuously to think over the procedures and criteria for regulatory decisions. They are

- changes in scientific understanding and techniques, as has been the case for example, with respect to acute toxicity assessment in recent years
- changes in society, i.e. in the perception by the public or by a majority or even by more or less important but concerned minorities, of what its needs are and of how they can best be satisfied

– changes in man's ability to affect himself and the living environment and in society's attitude towards that ability.

Legislation to protect public health and to prevent hazards to man and environment neither develops steadily nor in the same way in all fields. It rather advances in jumps in reaction to accidents, integrating and realizing scientific progress. The history of regulatory legislation on drugs and chemicals is a history of reactions to accidents. Because these regulations are concerned with protection they seem often to be negative and restrictive. But with growing knowledge and experience the requirements have to be readapted to match the need to allow decisions but not to hinder them.

That is what happens now with respect to acute toxicity assessment. Acute toxicity is a small part of the information scientists provide and regulators and physicians demand about medicines. It is of definite importance particularly in the early stage of development of a new drug. The evolution of toxicology has been clearly demonstrated here by the speakers, as they have shown the past and the present approaches to assessment of acute toxicity.

The results yielded by single dose toxicity experiments are the more useful the less they are gained in a – let me say – bureaucratic manner, as is the case in the classical formal LD50 test. It has been shown that the formal LD50 test is essentially a reduction of information expressing a complex situation in one (pseudo) exact figure. It was the unequivocal opinion of this conference that better observation – including behavioral aspects – of fewer animals can yield more and more useful information. An analysis of effects is more worthwhile than mere counting of end points. It makes more sense to study toxic effects rather than simply to record death. Hence toxicology comes back to its beginning of acute toxicity assessment, in which few animals were intensively observed until, after some decades the attitude had changed and large numbers of animals were sacrificed and almost only end points counted. Now we see a renaissance of skilled observation of a few animals with a minimum of distress and a sequential dose approach which again allows us to reduce the number of animals. And there is also hope that *in vitro* procedures, which today are mainly used to give complementary, additional data to those coming from animal experiments, can in the long run replace at least in part animal experiments for certain purposes. The search for alternative procedures to replace animal experiments is worldwide.

The more flexible approach to the assessment of acute toxicity needs more knowledge, more experience and more courage on both sides, on the side of industry as well as on the side of government and regulatory agencies. Both sides seem to be prepared for the task and the challenge.

We heard so from industry representatives yesterday and again right now in IFPMA's position paper. And in contrast to a widespread scepticism, drug control bodies worldwide do have an open and flexible approach.

The EC notes for guidance do not mention the LD50 any more; as a matter of fact one reason to revise the notes for guidance for single dose toxicity was to eliminate the requirement for formal LD50 tests. To follow the EC notes for guidance means to obtain more and better information using approximately 10% of the number of animals necessary for classical LD50 tests.

The US FDA position is similar in principle; a maximal amount of information should be obtained with a minimal number of animals. LD50 tests, with the exception of cytotoxic antitumour agents, are not directly or indirectly required; in-house workshops will ensure that they also will not be required in practice.

The exception is Japan. Here formal LD50 tests in rodents are still required at present, as well as single dose toxicity experiments yielding an estimate of that dose in dogs or monkeys. However, we are encouraged that the Japanese authorities were prepared to discuss their views at this meeting, listen to the debate we have had on scientific and ethical aspects and consider change.

The programme of this conference includes not only the assessment of acute toxicity in the development of new drugs but also in the characterisation of new industrial chemicals. The rationale was probably to proceed to questioning the importance of LD50 tests in the latter area once the problem has been settled for medicines. This is a justified reflection. So far the classification of chemicals is done worldwide according to LD50 values with somewhat different limits in the EC/OECD, USA, Japan and some other countries. But reconsideration of the sense of this kind of classification is evidently under way.

In organising this meeting IFPMA, together with BPI and ABPI, recognised and acknowledged a real problem. It was time to discuss this subject and I think the results are valuable. I come back to what I began with: If we can do better than we did in the past, let's do it!!

Subject Index

Acute Drug Overdose in Man 34
Acute toxicity testing
  ethical aspects 89
  factors influencing the results 14
  practical constraints 93
  regulatory constraints 95
  regulatory view in Japan 74
  scientific constraints 91
Alternative methodology 84
Alternatives to Animals in Toxicological Assessment 81
American Association for Accreditation of Laboratory Animal Care (AAALAC) 70
Analysis of protocol types 27
Animal Welfare Act 70
Antidepressants 36, 37
Antidote 14, 25

Behavioral signs 19
Bioavailability 25
Biologicals 91

Center for Devices and Radiological Health (CDRH) 67
Center for Drugs and Biologics (CDB) 67
Center for Food Safety and Applied Nutrition (CFSAN) 66
Center for Veterinary Medicine (CVM) 66
Chemical industry 20
Classification 12, 40
Committee for Proprietary Medicinal Products (CPMP) 55
Committee of Experts on the Transport of Dangerous Goods 59
Comparison of LD50 with experience in man 36
Confidence limits 12
Council Recommendation 83/571/EEC 56
Criteria for the classification of substances 24
Criteria for Toxicity Classification 29
Criticism of Current Practice 8
Cytotoxicity 49

Decision on the Mutual Acceptance of Data 83
Design of acute toxicity experiments 91
Dose levels 6

EC Directives 65/65 and 75/318 53
EC Note for Guidance 61
ECETOC 21
EEC/CPMP 55
Ethical aspects of acute toxicity testing 89

FDA 44
Federal Health Office of the Federal Republic of Germany 55
Formal LD50 97
Functional signs of toxicity 6

Guidelines to minimize the testing and use of animals 66

History 10

IFPMA view 96
In vitro alternatives to in vivo methodologies 68
In vitro methods 97
In vitro models 46
In vitro screening tests 84
Industrial chemicals 22
Intensive observation 17
International regulations 85

John Hopkins Center for Alternatives to Animal Testing 48

LC50 12
Legislation 23
Levels of Regulation 55
Limit dose 28
Limit test 44, 83, 97

Median lethal dose 5
Mefenamic acid 37
Minimal lethal dose 5

Subject Index

Modified LD50 tests 28
Morality of experiments that involve animals 89
Mutual Acceptance of Data 81

National Center for Toxicological Research (NCTR) 68
Non-steroidal anti-inflammatory drugs 36
Notes for Guidance 56
Notification No. 118, Pharmaceutical Affairs Bureau, Ministry of Health and Welfare 75
Numbers of animals 28

Observation 17, 91
OECD 41, 81, 82
OECD Chemicals Programme and Animal Welfare 81
OECD protocol 26
Organ specific toxicity 51
Outline protocol 21
Overdosage 15

Peri-lethal effects 24
Pesticide 25
Pharmaceutical Industry 42, 96

Pharmaceutical Manufacturers Association 43
Pharmaceuticals 11, 96
Phenylbutazone 37
Poison Control Center 34
Purpose of acute toxicity studies 57
Purposes of Acute Toxicity Testing 7

Range-finding 28
Re-evaluation 20
Recommendations 98
Reduction of suffering 8
Reference or Orientation Protocols 31
Registration 57
Regulations 7
Regulatory guidelines 20
Revision of Directive 75/318/EEC Part 2, Chapter 1, B. Toxicity 60

Safety standards 24
Side effects 14
Synergism 25

Up-down test 25, 44, 97
US/FDA View 65